D0836936

LIVING THE JOURNEY™

Also by Brandon Bays

The Journey

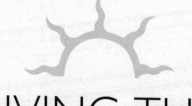

LIVING THE JOURNEY™

Using The Journey Method™ to Heal Your Life and Set Yourself Free

International Bestselling Author of *The Journey*™

Brandon Bays

Edited by Patricia Kendall, PhD, and Lesley Strutt, PhD

ATRIA PAPERBACK

New York   London   Toronto   Sydney   New Delhi

ATRIA PAPERBACK

A Division of Simon & Schuster, Inc.
1230 Avenue of the Americas
New York, NY 10020

Copyright © 2012 by Brandon Bays
Foreword © 2012 by Brandon Bays

All rights reserved, including the right to reproduce this book or portions thereof in any form whatsoever. For information address Atria Books Subsidiary Rights Department, 1230 Avenue of the Americas, New York, NY 10020

First Atria Paperback edition August 2012

ATRIA PAPERBACK and colophon are trademarks of Simon & Schuster, Inc.

For information about special discounts for bulk purchases, please contact Simon & Schuster Special Sales at 1-866-506-1949 or business@simonandschuster.com.

The Simon & Schuster Speakers Bureau can bring authors to your live event. For more information or to book an event contact the Simon & Schuster Speakers Bureau at 1-866-248-3049 or visit our website at www.simonspeakers.com.

Manufactured in the United States of America

10   9   8   7   6   5   4   3   2   1

Library of Congress Cataloging-in-Publication Data

Bays, Brandon.
   Living The Journey : using the journey method to heal your life and set yourself free / by Brandon Bays ; edited by Patricia Kendall and Lesley Strutt.—1st Atria pbk. ed.
     p. cm.
   "Atria non fiction original trade"—T.p. verso.
   1. Bays, Brandon. Journey. 2. Spiritual healing. I. Kendall, Patricia, PhD. II. Strutt, Lesley. III. Title.
   BL65.M4B395 2012
   616.99'400922—dc23
   [B]
                            2012007662

ISBN 978-1-4516-6562-8
ISBN 978-1-4516-6566-6 (ebook)

In gratitude to the healing grace pervading all of life.

May we all experience the magnificence
of our own souls.

Contents

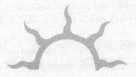

Foreword

This book arrived unexpectedly, as an answer to an innocent prayer I put out while sitting around the luncheon table with some Journey Practitioners at Life Transformation week in Denver in 2009.

I was sharing some particularly heartwarming healing stories of people I'd met around the world—stories of ordinary, everyday people who had experienced seemingly impossible healing in their lives, through using The Journey Method™.

Ten years ago, a woman came to the Journey Intensive in London with crippling multiple sclerosis. She sat in her wheelchair drooling, having been told she would never heal. Ten years later she bounded up on stage to let everyone know she was now a marathon runner. Although she was a decade older than when I had first met her, she looked ten years younger—so fresh and alive. She admonished us all to "Keep doing your Journeys!"

Another woman at an intro talk in Cheltenham, UK, shared that she had tried every healing modality for her frozen back, both medical and complementary. She had been in excruciating pain for seven years, and after three operations, her doctors had said there was simply nothing more they could do for her. After just two Journey processes with a Journey Practitioner, not only did her frozen back heal, but her arm, which she had not been able to raise above her waistline, could now extend over her head. She waved it proudly to show us all.

Then I shared the story of a seventeen-year-old girl from New Zealand who was given a grave prognosis: she only had a short time left to live. She had three inoperable, untreatable brain tumors, and she decided to use The Journey process from *The Journey* book every week. After one year, her MRI scans showed no tumors.

One story that really blew me away was that of a fifty-year-old woman from Israel who contracted polio at age seven and as a result had a crooked, crippled body and one leg significantly shorter than the other. After going through the year-long Journey Practitioner Program, she had not only healed her life, but her shorter leg grew by 5 centimeters (a bit less than 2 inches). Her body became straight and whole. Her leg grew in her fifties! What an astounding healing experience.

I am always truly awed by the body's capacity to heal, even against seemingly impossible odds. Physical healing stories from people using The Journey Method are endless—such a vision of possibility for us all. Over the last seventeen years of giving Journey seminars, sometimes traveling to thirty-five countries a year, I have personally witnessed thousands of these healings and have received tens of thousands of emails, letters and communications that confirm our body's immense potential to heal. It never ceases to inspire me—this miraculous healing intelligence that exists within us—how the body seems capable of healing just about anything, any physical challenge, illness or injury. And it is a source of constant wonder to me that in fact the body is *designed* to heal. It's a healing machine!

But what really breaks my heart open is when people heal their *lives*, how, even in the most adverse circumstances, the human heart triumphs. It awes me to see the strength and courage of the human spirit and its capacity to heal seemingly unbearable, insurmountable conditions. I am deeply humbled by the nobility of heart, the courage of someone to open their heart, even after the trauma and shutdown following rape or abuse. I'm stunned by whatever determination it must require to face down and clear forty years of debilitating, unrelenting depression. I am freshly astounded by the human heart's ability to forgive even the unforgiveable—the war trauma, the loss and the devastation of losing one's entire family. And still somehow, the largeness, the magnificence of the human spirit is such that it simply will not be crushed. It triumphs even in the most adverse, heartbreaking of circumstances.

And I feel deep, deep gratitude for the power of the Journey tools, these practical methods that give people the ability to finish with their painful stories and to open into the natural joy, the love, the authentic greatness that is our own essence.

After all these years, what is clearer to me now than ever before, is that when there is a strong prayer and the openness to embark on your own healing journey, to dive in and meet your deepest fears, to welcome your deepest pain—when there is the willingness to fully use this powerful, liberating process work—it is possible to clear even the most deeply held cell memories, the most difficult challenges, even when life says it's not possible. Healing is available to us all. Not only is it possible, it is within all of our reach.

The truth is, you can heal any aspect of your life.

So as I was sitting at that table with my colleagues, my fellow Journey Practitioners, I put out an innocent prayer that someone would gather together some of these stories—stories of ordinary, everyday people who had experienced extraordinary healing. I wished someone would compile them and then share with our world these simple but heartfelt journeys of healing and awakening.

Pat Kendall, who was sitting next to me, heard this simple wish, and something entered her heart. Her hair stood on end, and she felt a deep pull from within, a call to answer this prayer, to gather healing stories that we could all relate to, that we could see ourselves in—real stories of real human beings who experienced the same heartbreak, loss, abuse, depression, addiction, anger or shutdown that we have all experienced. Stories from people who cleared unhealthy beliefs, liberated themselves from unrelenting life circumstances, overcame insurmountable conditions; people who experienced years of relationship problems yet still found their way home to the joy, the freedom, the love that is the essence of all of us.

And so together she and her editing partner Lesley Strutt collected, compiled and edited these life-transforming stories—true stories that will not only heal your life but will open the door for *you* to begin your own healing journey.

When I first read these stories, I laughed, I cried, my heart broke wide open, and something in me opened up to a deeper level of healing. I saw myself in these stories and was moved by the naked, raw exposure from which these authors wrote. I saw my life mirrored in their journeys. For me reading the whole book turned out to be an odyssey of clearing blocks, releasing shutdowns, letting go of the hurts, pain and anger that I had stored inside. I felt the truth of what they shared resonate within my own heart and underwent my own journey as I opened into the joy, the gratitude and the love that is the true and healing magnificence of the human heart.

After completing the book, I realized that you would feel the same pull from within that I did: an invitation—indeed, an imperative—to go on your own healing journey. I knew that you would want to respond to that pull by experiencing The Journey Method yourself. So I offered to put a Journey Process into the back of this book, one specifically designed for it, so you could roll up *your* sleeves and begin your journey in freedom and awaken to your own greatness. I wanted you to have the gift of living life from the love in your heart, from the truth of who you really are.

My prayer is that not only will you feel inspired by these moving stories, you will also feel compelled to *do* something about it—that they will catalyze you to begin your own healing journey.

So who is the real author of this book? Life itself. Truth itself. And yet with all my heart, I would like to thank all the contributors who opened up their hearts, exposed their lives and took us on their journeys with them into the love and joy that is our essence. What a generous offering, a courageous, priceless offering.

And heartfelt gratitude to Pat and Lesley for offering this immense labor of love to life. They pored over every word to ensure the stories were clear and potent. They, too, share my prayer that you will be inspired by these life-transforming stories, and that these journeys will catalyze you to embark on *your* journey, to heal and transform *your* life.

Let this book be your invitation to heal your life and set yourself free.

Namaste,
Brandon

LIVING THE
JOURNEY™

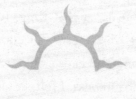

I

One Crumb at a Time

by Debbie Clarke

Change . . . it's something that can occur in the blink of an eye, or it can be something that happens so slowly that it's not until you wake up one day and ask, "How did I get here?" that you even notice the change. This can be either change for the better or for the worse, on the scale of, How's your life working for you?

My experience of change has been the slow, subtle type. It wasn't until my life had tipped to a very low point that I woke up and began to realize that I couldn't continue on the path I was on. Even my awakening to the fact of how bad I felt was slow. It was as if I couldn't have tolerated noticing it all at once, so I become aware of each aspect, one little bit at a time.

Let me describe what my life was like back in October 2006. I was a month away from turning forty-six years old, and I was in a longtime relationship with my spouse, Dan.

We had just celebrated twenty-four years of being together, and our relationship had grown unhappy and unhealthy in many ways. In my eyes, at that time, it was all because of Dan. I blamed Dan's discontent, his choices, his moods and unhappiness as being the cause of our problems and ultimately my own unhappiness. I felt so sad most of the time, as well as alone, isolated, stressed, frustrated, hopeless and unloved; the list was endless.

To make matters worse, I had been diagnosed with rheumatoid arthritis nineteen years earlier. This disease had, at times rapidly and more often slowly and insidiously, accelerated to the point that eventually I was no longer able to work. Despite the evidence that something was very wrong, though, I had lived in denial from the time I had first gotten sick.

My jaw was the first area to be affected. Within two months I couldn't open my mouth more than enough to fit my baby finger between my top and bottom teeth. I would force myself to go to work every day, and I remember that, while sitting at my desk, it would take me the entire morning to eat a muffin, one crumb at a time.

Surgery repaired my jaw somewhat, but then the disease began in earnest as one joint at a time began to inflame and swell. Soon my breastbone was swollen and protruding, and it felt like someone was sitting on my chest at all times. If I coughed or sneezed, the pain was unbelievable, almost as if someone had ripped me wide open. My shoulders were painful, and I couldn't reach over my head. In order to get myself out of bed in the morning, I would grab the front of my own pajamas and pull myself up. To wash my hair in the shower, I would need to bend forward and bring my head down to where I could reach my hair. Both of my knees ached, and I limped; my neck barely turned, and each movement of my head was agonizing. My low back was stiff and very painful. There were almost no spots on my body that didn't hurt. Each morning it was only after hours of struggle and incredible pain that I would be ready to start the trip to work via public transit.

I read an article once by a woman suffering from rheumatoid arthritis, and she said that her life was about planning. She had to preplan every step she took and every moment of her day. I had been doing exactly that, and such was the depth of my denial that I had not even been aware of it! I would plan ahead what hand I would hold on with when I boarded a bus, and make sure not to carry anything and always to have a hand free. I would pray that there would be a seat available, and one that I could get in and out of easily and not make a spectacle of myself.

As I write this now, I'm still amazed that even with all the pain and suffering that I endured, *not calling attention to myself* was foremost in my mind. I have to laugh, because the visual I have of a female version of the Tin Man of Oz making her way through her day and not calling attention to herself is so ridiculous. The good news is that most people around me were so "asleep" in their lives that they didn't notice me in mine.

Even when I did stop working, only my closest friends were even aware that there was anything wrong with me. People who worked beside me every day had no idea. I was the master of disguise. I kept a smile on my face and hid my pain, because that is what I believed I was supposed to do.

I was the consummate people pleaser and had to give 150 percent at work and be the best social worker ever. At home all I wanted was for Dan to be happy, because I believed if he was happy, then I would be. I ignored and denied my pain in an attempt to keep everyone else happy.

My family lived about four hours away, and I traveled there as much as I could, because I needed to be close to them and please them, too. I always felt split: there was my family and my life in my hometown, and there was Dan and my life in Toronto. Whenever I was with my family, I felt I should be with Dan, and when I was with Dan, I felt that my family needed me. I remember a toy called Stretch Armstrong that my nephew Keith had back in the '90s. The toy was made of a soft rubber; you could pull Stretch's arms, and they would extend to abnormal lengths. I see my face on the Stretch Armstrong toy, being pulled until my arms can stretch from Toronto to the Ottawa Valley. There is sadness here as I realize what I expected from my body, and yet I can laugh because it really is a funny visual.

It's all so obvious to me now that the outer struggles were being reflected in my body. Playing these games and using these strategies to fulfill myself—and looking outside of myself to others to give me value and meaning—was causing my joints and my body to be in a metaphorical tug-of-war that week by week, month by month was becoming physical. However, at that time I was so busy planning my every movement and just getting through my day that I couldn't see the big picture. I was like a workhorse wearing blinders and plodding along through what felt like wet concrete. I felt as if I carried the weight of the world on my shoulders. Every step and movement was a struggle.

I continued like this for thirteen years, until I needed to have a second surgery on my shoulder as well as surgery on both my knees. The doctor told me that they could do a few more surgeries and then they would need to start replacing my joints; but if the artificial joints wore out, there was nothing that could be done. It was all very difficult because I was so young. Usually people are getting joints replaced in their senior years, and I was only in my forties. The cold, hard truth finally hit me: my body was deteriorating, and I only had the one body. I had better wake up.

With a heavy heart and incredible fear I agreed to leave work. I will never forget the day that I read the doctor's report that my rheumatologist had completed in order for me to receive long-term disability benefits from my employer. I opened the envelope that he had given me and read "Permanently Disabled." I felt like someone had pulled the bottom out of my world.

At the time, I was sitting waiting to have my blood tests done, and as much as I wanted to sob like a baby, I felt I had to hold it together, just as I had always done. The technician called me in, and I stuffed that sadness down inside me and smiled brightly. When I got home, I cried to Dan, at first, but whenever I cried, it seemed to physically hurt him, so eventually I held it in.

My family was the same. I didn't want to worry them, and if I cried, they appeared to be so uncomfortable with my sadness. The worst thing for me is to see someone else uncomfortable. It was less painful to hold it inside than to risk making them feel uncomfortable.

I realize now that there was a deeper deterrent: I feared that if I dared allow that sadness, it would be like the Hoover Dam letting loose, and the tears would never stop. All I wanted was for people to be happy and have fun around me, and there's nothing that stops a party like someone crying an ocean of tears on you. I'm having another visual of the doll I used to have, one that you filled with water and it would cry and wet in the diaper. I see myself with my tear ducts releasing a never-ending stream of tears. That could get messy!

So at the age of forty I found myself unable to work, trapped in a body that the doctors predicted with certainty would slowly and steadily deteriorate. I was taking forty pills a week to manage my arthritis and the related conditions, such as stomach problems from the heavy-duty anti-inflammatory medication. At least once a week I would vomit in the middle of the night. One medication had the possible side effect of damaging my stomach lining and causing ulcers. Another medication could cause liver damage, and yet another could cause irreversible eye problems and loss of vision. The double-edged sword was that if I didn't take medication, I could not get out of bed. If I forgot to take my medication in the morning, then by noon I would start to feel my whole body becoming even more stiff and painful, and it would remind me to quickly take my pills. I cannot even fathom what my life would have been like without that medication.

I had always struggled with who I was, and when I worked, at least I knew myself as a social worker and had a purpose, a reason to get out of bed in the morning. Now who was I, with no career and no purpose? I felt worthless, weak and so afraid.

I looked to Dan to fill me up, and this caused him to pull further away. The desperate need was more than he could cope with. I felt like a victim, like this had happened *to* me, and each night I would pray to be stronger physically, emotionally and spiritually.

I began reading self-help New Age spirituality books and began journaling. I took a meditation course and spent the next six years searching for answers to what had gone wrong in my life, wanting someone or something to fix it.

I remember in the summer of 2006, I picked up a book by Doreen Virtue, who does Angel Readings and connects with angels as guides. In this particular book, Doreen was writing about her life of traveling, doing workshops and attending spiritual events and ceremonies. I said out loud to anyone that would listen, "This is the life I want." I felt it resonated so strongly in every fiber of my being; I had never experienced such certainty about anything in my life.

Of course, my mind checked in with its fear, doubt and judgment, and it started to question how this could be possible. Who did I think I was, comparing myself to the likes of Doreen Virtue? My mind was successful in having me doubt myself, and yet for a few moments I had really felt a glimmer of excitement and hope in my body.

My interest was piqued, and a few months later my sister and I went for an Angel Reading in Ottawa. I was told that my angels were showing the reader that I would be a coach for women and children; she asked me if I had ever heard of The Journey.

I came back home to Toronto and checked the Journey website. As grace would have it, there was a Journey Intensive weekend in Toronto a few weeks later. Dan and I went together to the weekend, and I immediately knew that this was what I had been searching for. Here were the tools to tap into my own body wisdom; and that's where I found the "ME" I had seemingly lost connection with.

When we were instructed to find a partner to do this process with, I immediately panicked, and the old fear of being picked last rose up in my mind. Again grace guided me, this time to turn to the wonderful soul next to me, named Sheila. Together we guided each other through our first Journey process. We instantly connected, and the next spring we traveled together to complete all the courses in the Practitioner Program. This is when I realized that when you open your heart and speak truth, you connect to people at a deeper level, through truth, and I immediately formed a connection with another being in a way that previously would have taken me years to develop.

During that first weekend I did two processes that both took me into a deeper consciousness and into my internal body wisdom. My experience has been that when I do work at this deeper place, it is difficult to recall the details of the process. I will explain what occurred as best I can.

In most of our Journey processes, our body wisdom allows us to feel an emotion and then takes us back to a time when we first felt that emotion. The emotion I felt then was a blend of fear and anxiety, and the memory that came was when I was about seven years old, playing outside. One of my siblings came running outside and said that our dad was freaking out. We all ran inside, and I remember that he was yelling at my mom, who was standing wordlessly listening and watching him as he yelled and cursed and kicked the cupboard door and picked up the end of the table and dropped it again. He banged the table and counter with his fist and kicked and roared some more. I stood in the doorway, frozen in fear and yet somehow forced to watch. It was like seeing an accident on the side of the road and not being able to look away.

I believe this was the first time I had ever seen my dad so angry, and I was confused and afraid and curious as to what had happened, and angry at him for scaring me and for scaring my mom. (I don't know if she was afraid, but that is what the younger me thought.) I later realized that I also took on a belief at that time: If you didn't control your anger, you could scare people, or people would think there was something wrong with you. I also later discovered that right then I made a vow never to show anger.

In my process, when I invited my dad to sit with me at a campfire of unconditional love and acceptance, I was able to tell him exactly how this made me feel. I was able to see the pattern that I developed to never do anything to upset my dad for fear of a reenactment of this scene. I was also able to speak to my mom, and I realized there was anger at her for never speaking up for herself and for never teaching or encouraging *me* to speak up for *myself*.

The beauty of this process was that in it both my mom and my dad had an opportunity to respond and explain to me what they were feeling. My dad was a truck driver, and every week he was on the road from Sunday evening until late the following Friday night. He was home with us for less than two days every week. When I saw how he felt like an outsider in his own home, I felt a newfound compassion for him. I also saw how my mom was exactly the same as me; all she wanted was for people to be happy, and she did that by always complying and pleasing others and never making waves. They both were doing the best they could with the emotional understanding and resources they had at the time.

I honestly can't recall the second process that I experienced that weekend; all I know is that something shifted inside of me. I walked away on Sunday night feeling so peaceful, aware that a memory that I had stored for forty years could be looked at with clarity; it could be changed, I could forgive them both for their actions, and I could forgive that younger me for creating my own pain about the memory and the people involved.

Within the first week following the Journey Intensive weekend, Dan and I sat down to talk. He told me that he could see I was in a "good place" and that he felt our relationship had run its course and that we should go our separate ways. I calmly replied, "Okay," and it honestly was okay. This, coming from a person who had done everything to hang on to Dan, as he did everything to push me away! The more he had pushed, the more I hung on. I had made my life around Dan and had no idea who I was without him. Dan is such a big, beautiful personality, and I had identified myself through him for twenty-four years.

I am still in awe that one weekend at the Journey Intensive shifted something in me and created a knowing: that this was the right thing to do. In that moment all fear fell away, and there was only peace and acceptance.

Dan and I cried many times about the loss of the good parts of our relationship, and Dan said more than once, "I don't know why I am doing this." I truly believe that on some level he did it for me. I know that I could not have done what I have done or experienced what I have experienced, if Dan and I were still together. I needed to break free of the codependency that we had created in order to find my own path.

I went on with my Journeywork, completed the Practitioner Program and qualified as an Accredited Journey Practitioner. I then completed the Visionary Leadership and Conscious Coaching Programs, and the awareness, growth and emotional and physical healing have continued.

These past six years, Dan and I have remained friends. This transition has at times been painful as I let go of Dan and the old patterns. Dan has been a wonderful teacher for me, and each time I am triggered by something that he does or says, it shows me what I need to look at within myself. Many times when I have returned from a Journey event where I have gained new insights, I will contact Dan and say,

"I am so sorry for the times that I blamed you for my pain." It feels so liberating to be able to cut the energetic cord to that old hurt and pain and the victim story that I told myself. I realize it was my pain that I projected and blamed on him; when I acknowledge and accept that pain, that is when the healing can occur.

My physical health has improved dramatically. I cannot pinpoint one process or Journey event to which I can attribute my physical healing. When I clear out old pain and hurt, as I "let go," my body slowly responds as well.

I do recall a couple of incidents that left me in awe: the improvement was very obvious, without a doubt. The first "before and after" scenario involved the morning yoga I participated in at two different Journey events. I had never done yoga before because it was such a challenge for me to get down on the floor and stand back up with the limited movement that I had. However, I was willing to participate and do what I could. At the first retreat, Manifest Abundance, in April 2007, I remember vividly that at one point I was attempting to do a Downward Dog pose, leaning over with hands and feet on the floor, and my right wrist wouldn't bend, so I made a fist and used the side of my hand to support myself.

When I attended the No Ego retreat three months later, I was again participating in morning yoga. We did the Downward Dog pose, and at first I didn't notice, but then I realized that my wrist was bent and both palms were flat on the floor. My eyes welled up with tears, because this was the first time in years I had experienced physical improvement.

The second step forward happened at another weekend retreat, called Healing with Conscious Communication, also in April 2007. On Saturday afternoon during a break, we went outside to enjoy the sunshine. The only place to sit was on the curb of the driveway beside the hotel, so my friends all crouched down and sat on the curb. I considered it but knew that there was no way for me to bend enough to get down there and even less possibility of getting back up. I remained standing.

On Sunday, we did the same, only this time I looked down and thought, "I can do this." So I turned and sat down. I was thrilled. I said to my friends, "I sat down!" They were a little perplexed by this seemingly obvious statement. "You have no idea. I haven't been able to do this in over twenty years!" Then I was able to get back up on my feet again. It truly was a miracle! Sometime in the previous twenty-four hours, my body had become less rigid and allowed me to bend and sit on the curb in the beautiful sunshine with my friends.

I have realized so many things, and the biggest one is how I had lived in my head, as if my body was just along for the ride. I see how I always hated my body and felt that it was unattractive. I recall at the age of eight, I thought I looked fat in a swimsuit, was self-conscious about my body and kept it covered. I took my body for granted, didn't listen to it and totally disconnected from it. I see how it rebelled against me, and how I rebelled in a quiet and self-destructive way against myself. The arthritis was my way of expressing the anger that I so long ago had vowed never to express. It was me screaming a big "Fuck you!" internally, and the fire in my inflamed joints was certainly a testament to that. No one got hurt except for me, and the rage got to be released internally rather than externally.

It has been over four years since my first Journey weekend, and my life has been forever changed. It has been an incredible time of opportunities and experiences that I had never thought possible. From the moment that I decided to follow this path, everything has been unfolding as though divinely guided. I had the realization just a few days ago that my life is easy and effortless until *I* decide that it's not; then *I* can make it a struggle. When I become aware of the struggle and again let go and allow the magic, the easy and effortless life appears again.

It is truly empowering to know that I can decide how I want my life to look and feel. I used to say, "I have to," and now I say, "I choose to." I'm not saying that it's always easy; everyday life offers a double bind, or two ends of that proverbial tug-of-war rope, that I can choose to pick up and pull, or I can just notice and allow the emotions to present themselves. By "double bind," I mean the simultaneous "I want to" and "I don't want to," the "I should" and "I shouldn't," "I could" and "I couldn't," "I have to" . . . the list goes on and on. I don't know about you, but for me these binds are exhausting, energy stealing and mind-boggling. I understand that this is the cost our ego exacts, and that heart, mind, left brain, right brain can choose to work in harmony or in disharmony. And I have found some techniques that are very effective for me to regain this harmony within.

One day I was at my sister's house doing my income tax.

However, I couldn't concentrate, and I was having sciatic pain down my leg. I tried to keep working and ignore it and it got worse. Finally I stopped and asked, "What's here?" and instantly I realized that I was feeling guilty. I had left my dad at home, and he had wanted me to take him out for a drive, and here I was doing something for myself. The moment I named it and acknowledged the guilt, the pain went away, and I was able to focus and get clarity to do what I needed to do.

The same is true for any physical pain in my body. I had suffered from huge, painful cold sores on my lip in the past. Now as soon as I feel one starting, I go right into the consciousness of the cold sore and ask, "What's here?" or "If there were words or emotions inside, what might they be?" Every time it has been unexpressed anger, and by allowing and acknowledging it, the cold sore never develops. I usually either say the words out loud or journal. I write, "I am angry that . . ." and fill in the blank or blanks. This also has worked for a sore throat that I am usually convinced is a cold starting. Every time it has been unexpressed anger, and when expressed, the sore throat is gone the next day.

This is such a gift that I have given myself. To be able to reconnect to my body and really listen to it is amazing. As I said earlier, my physical health has vastly improved. Under my doctor's supervision I have recently reduced my medication down to nothing. That's right—I went from forty pills a week for my arthritis down to zero. I am left with the damage in my joints that occurred when my joints were inflamed, and each day I trust that they will continue to heal. My neck is still stiff and my arms cannot (yet) extend over my head. And if bending forward to wash my hair in the shower is the toughest thing I have to face, I will accept it with love.

I have made peace with my body and with the rheumatoid arthritis. I am truly grateful for everything that has happened to me and for every pain I have felt. If that was what was needed for me to wake up and pay attention to my body and my life, then I am eternally thankful for all of it. I am now practicing being accepting of my body, just the way it is. I want to honor my body by eating to nourish it, as opposed to filling it to avoid hunger, to comfort myself or to avoid feeling an emotion.

I believe that every situation that comes to me is an opportunity to learn and grow, and when I step out of my comfort zone, any hidden limiting beliefs or triggers are revealed to me. The way that I lived my life before was to deny and avoid and put up a false front. I also looked outside myself for happiness. I pretended that I was fine and that my life was great. I hid my physical and emotional pain, and when Dan and I separated, except for a few close people who knew the truth, most people in our life were shocked, as they thought everything was wonderful between us. The fact that I am sharing my truth in full exposure here is a testament to the power of this work. I choose to live in truth, and when I open and expose, it gives me a connection to myself. All that I searched for outside myself is here within me.

I truly love this work and believe in it. I lately have had the great honor of sharing this work with others and traveling from Labrador to British Columbia and many places in between. I have been able to participate in sweat lodge ceremonies and meet and learn from the wisdom of the First Nations people. Magically, I am living the life that Doreen Virtue described in her book. Somehow my dream was sent out into this generous and loving Universe, and it came back to me easily and effortlessly.

My family has been a true blessing to me; they have never stopped loving me. I never had my own children, and my nieces and nephews have been a true light in my life. I joke that I am busy spending their inheritance, with all my traveling and Journey courses; and all kidding aside, the best gift I can give them is not money. The greatest legacy I can pass down is to walk the walk and show them that life is to be lived and embraced.

When my aunt Florence was near the end of her life and reliant on an oxygen machine to breathe, she told my sister and me as we were leaving, "Live your life to the fullest." That is my intention: to live my life fully and to share these tools with others, so that they can choose to do the same.

The greatest gift that The Journey and Visionary Leadership have given me is awareness: awareness that I create my own reality and that I have the ability to change my life and heal my body. And I have! As I have opened in this awareness, the rheumatoid arthritis that once held me captive has loosened its grip. As I welcome long-suppressed emotions and uncover and clear limiting beliefs, my body thanks me by moving more freely. Hope replaces hopelessness and trust replaces fear. I have gone from a life that was filled with emotional and physical pain that made every day a struggle to a life filled with possibilities, ease, excitement and so much gratitude.

I have been fortunate to have longtime friends who bring me so much joy, laughter and love. And the new friends I have made through The Journey have opened my heart even wider. If you see me now, I will likely be smiling, only now it's a real smile, not a mask for the pain. As I write, there are tears here that flow freely, and they are tears of joy.

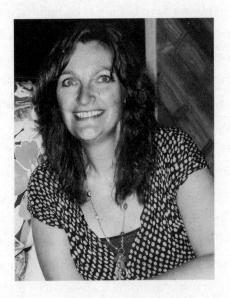

Debbie Clarke *lives in Toronto and is an Accredited Journey Practitioner and Visionary Leadership Coach. She has spent the past few years focusing on her own healing. An important aspect of this healing has been to support Journey and Visionary Leadership work across Canada. Debbie can be contacted at debbieclarke5075@sympatico.ca.*

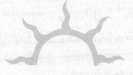

2

The Good Little Girl

by Patricia Kendall

The Black Cloud was clever. Like a stray cat that roams the edges of the backyard for weeks, then ventures closer and closer to the house before finally dashing into the warm basement, the Cloud had haunted the edges of my childhood for almost a decade. Biding its time, awaiting the perfect, predestined moment, it would slither through the back of my mind when a friend did not invite me to her party, or when my mother would make me the butt of one of her crushing "jokes." I would sense the dragging of my thoughts, a whisper of unease, a hint of despair like a dark gray cloth thrown carelessly over my brightest moments.

Good Little Girls, however, are Cheerful. So I would skitter away into a brave smile, into the nearest book or project: doing something, anything, to help me ignore the vast, alien, brooding presence that lay like a fog bank on the horizon of my mind. I would run, run, run away into the exciting lives of book heroes and heroines, the beauty and fascination of my glorious green West Coast world, the ceaseless striving and dutiful accomplishments of the Good Little Girl, Smart Student, Dutiful Daughter, who could always be counted on to Do It Right . . .

Then, one soggy Vancouver afternoon as I wound my way home through the darkening, glistening streets, with a stick in my hand chattering through the wrought-iron railings of fence post after fence post, the Black Cloud pounced. One moment I was fifteen, bouncing home from a babysitting afternoon, the ever-present zipped binder of schoolbooks banging on my hip in thumping counterpoint to the clatter of fence-and-stick—and the next moment I was no age at all. I was, in fact, no longer a human being. I was in—no, I *was*—a black, tarry mass of unfathomable pain, utter despair and complete inertia.

I put down the stick, carefully (Good Little Girls are Careful). The bookbinder slid down my leg. My knees melted into the rain, and I found myself sitting on the waterlogged lawn of someone else's house. I could not move. I could not think. I could not speak. I did not wish to speak, or move or think. If there was an "I" it wished only to die.

Much, much later in what then passed for my life, I realized that the Black Cloud descended every three years for a few months, then gradually picked up and moved on (leaving its bags and numerous calling cards, however) until the next triennial visit. I remember sitting in my high school classes (Good Little Girls get Straight A's) with unbidden tears running down my cheeks, utterly mortified yet physically unable to open my mouth and answer the teacher's anxious questions. I remember the bright promise of my summer in France turning to wintry darkness as I sought shelter in church after church after church, wearing out my knees on the stone floors, praying for something, anything, to keep me from hell here and now—and having my first bout of the ulcerative colitis that dogged me for the following forty years. I remember graduating from college top in my class (Good Little Girls get Scholarships) and standing before the Faculty Club fireplace in my long white dress like a wedding gown, carrying a dozen long-stemmed red roses, smiling stiffly at the faculty members who had lined up to honor me and congratulate me on the bright promise of my academic career. And hearing over and over in my head, "Dust and ashes. Dust and ashes. Dust and ashes." I can still taste them, those ashes in my mouth and in my heart.

Of course, I turned to Good Little Girl strategies to help me run from the Black Cloud. Alcohol and drugs were Bad Little Girl strategies; I didn't use them. But losing myself in book after book after book kept me quiet, isolated and out of the present moment. Getting good grades in school, college, graduate school kept my mind spinning fast enough to dull the pain. (Great discovery: you can't think and feel at the same time!) And finding someone to love and marry me helped me ignore the hissing flames of hell yawning at my feet. Doing Everything for Everyone, espousing causes, helping the poor, the uneducated, the outcast kids and just plain miserable adults, might possibly allow me to work off some of my eternal debt to God, to the Universe, to Life itself. I poured my love into everything I could—except myself. Myself I hated. I cowered eternally under the unending, scathing, shaming criticism of the Voice, which, unlike the Cloud, didn't ever go away. But Good Little Girls Never Rebel, so I put up with the Voice because it—so it said—was the only thing that could keep me Good.

Unfortunately, these strategies weren't free of charge. In fact, they cost me just about everything I had ever cherished, as I turned into a little tin soldier mechanically marching off to war against poverty and illiteracy, against discrimination and abuse, never noticing that while I was *against* a lot, there didn't seem to be much that I was really *for*. My old beliefs in God had had to be thrown out—too narrow—and though atheism or at least agnosticism was the only thing that made sense, it also made me miserable. Now I dreamed of standing outside the doors of churches: beautiful music floated out, but I was barred from entering. I was in a constant state of homesickness, without even knowing what Home was or where. I tried two cults, divorce, another marriage. I helped raise five teenagers. I taught disadvantaged kids of all kinds. I turned my hand to art, my voice to music. I wrote shining, luminous articles in magazines and journals and then returned to my shaking, anxious, angry life.

On my fortieth birthday, a few months into my second marriage, I made a vow to myself that I would be true to the Truth, wherever I found it. Surely that would please whatever gods there were! And the very next day, while jogging along the sidewalk (Good Little Girls Stay in Shape), I found myself veering over into the road, hoping a car would run over me and just end it. The colitis was gaining ground, and I had added mononucleosis to the mix. My son had left the family. Even my students, who had once loved me, now appeared to despise me. It felt as if I had experienced nothing but heartbreak and blame: in my original family, in all my relationships with men, in all my business ventures and careers, even in the various religious groups and cults I had tried. And every three years the Black Cloud would descend even lower.

I wanted out, and that scared me. So I tried getting some help for this awful self, this miserable creature who, it appeared from the feedback I got, was "too" everything. Too emotional, too rigid. Too sad, too angry. Too driven, too lazy. Too vocal, too silent. Too smart, too dumb. Too active, too passive. Too much . . . and much, much too little.

The first psychologist told me, after fifteen minutes, that I had to decide if I wanted to stay in my marriage and act like a five-year-old or get out and grow up. I got out. Of his office. The second put me on drugs. I took one dose of the "calming meds" and went right off the deep end: paranoid, hallucinating, nearly catatonic with terror. I gave up on doctors and grimly struggled on. My blood sugar began to swing wildly, and I developed allergies to every foodstuff I put into my body. I barely slept at all. And, Good Little Tin Soldier, I kept marching.

I left the school district and, eventually, my marriage. I helped found an organizational development consulting company. (Perhaps influencing "the many" would work better than teaching "the few.") The company flourished; I didn't. I was now working more than one hundred hours a week, writing speeches for air force generals and then the joint chiefs of staff, creating all the materials for our many courses and teaching some of them myself. And my body and heart suffered, and suffered. By now I had pain in all eighteen of the body points indicative of fibromyalgia, but I didn't see a doctor. I had given up on doctors, and Good Little Girls are Consistent. I would have a sinus infection for three weeks, have two weeks of respite, then back would come the same virulent infection. My car was rear-ended seven times, and I sustained injury in the same shoulder each time. And then I very nearly died of pneumonia. Gasping for breath, on fire with fever, coughing my lungs out, I sent out a cry for help: "Show me what to do! If this is wrong for me, show me what's right!"

Help came, though at first it wore the face of pain. Within weeks, I was thrown out of the company I had helped found and into which I had poured all my retirement funds. From one day to the next I had no job, no income, no colleagues. I had nothing left: no self-respect, no purpose in life, no strategies for escaping the yawning pit of hell. My new life partner had also been fired, and was as deeply hurt and confused as I, unable to help ease my suffering. And then . . .

One day I was in a chiropractor's office waiting to pick up some supplements. To pass the time and appease my reading addiction, I thumbed through a book of alternative healing modalities lying on the coffee table and was arrested by an article on hypnotherapy. I called the hypnotherapist and made an appointment—for my partner, of course, not myself. I didn't need help. My partner insisted I be present during her session; and before the session was over I knew this was my next step. As part of my contribution to the world, I had facilitated informal inner healing work with others for many years, often using the very same phrasing and imagery the hypnotherapist had used. I asked about possible training and enrolled in an extensive certification program. In the following months, I found and healed many of the causes of my inner pain and became moderately functional as a supposedly recovering workaholic. I opened my doors for business. I assisted many, many beautiful people to come out of deep physical and psychological trauma and reenter their worlds as productive, "well-adjusted" members of society. And yet I still yearned for Home. And the Black Cloud, while no longer as debilitating as before, still hovered . . .

In 2003, as I entered my tenth year of a successful psychotherapy practice, I felt restlessness in my bones. The Cloud swooped lower, muttering, and I felt the quicksands of lethargy sucking at my feet. Yes, using hypnotherapy, Cellular Release therapy, EMDR and other alternative modalities, I often witnessed deep physical and emotional healing. Yet satisfying as that was, I kept feeling I was ushering my clients to a door—the entrance to a place I had only glimpsed from afar, a haven of wholeness, delight and freedom—but was not able to conduct them through that door because I had not been through it myself. Desperate, thrashing in the tarry pool of my despair, I called out to I-knew-not-what: "Open this door to me!"

A week later a client dropped a book into my lap: *The Journey*, by Brandon Bays. Ten days after that I went to my first Journey Intensive weekend, swinging wildly between hope and doubt: Is this real, or is it a cult?

Made cult-savvy by painful experience, I was delighted to hear the presenter tell us immediately to "take out our BS detectors." (Mine was already out.) We were never told what to believe; facts were presented to our minds, experiences to our hearts and bodies. The conclusions were up to us. Were we willing to take a chance? To be led into the emotions we had all been running from, and through them to our Source, the essence of our being? Would we take the gamble of opening that door, of turning to face the tiger padding along behind us?

I turned. I opened to the feelings that had been chasing me. And behold, they were not my death bringers after all. They were my freedom! By Saturday evening, driving home as the sun poured glorious and golden over the distant Rockies, it felt to me as if the heavens had opened and I was, for the first time since the age of fifteen, truly at peace.

By the end of the seminar I knew this was truly life-bringing work, and my next step as a therapist. But what *was* the magic here? The format wasn't that different from what I had done for almost a decade as a hypnotherapist and EMDR clinician. Yet these simple processes brought me a gift beyond all possibility: freedom from the tyranny of "my story" and how it had laid waste to my body and my life, tearing happiness to shreds and turning success to ashes, ashes, ashes; release from the blocks and beliefs that had prevented natural healing and a true homecoming to myself.

The difference seemed to lie in who or what was *running*

the process—and that weekend showed me the difference via a close-to-home example. By 2003, my ulcerative colitis, that painful bleeding of the intestinal lining that had first shown up in France when I was twenty-one, had defied all healing modalities for forty years. The hypnotherapist and I, for example, would agree to "go into" the colon to see what was going on there and ask the colon how to heal it. Or, the EMDR clinician and I would list and desensitize traumatic events that might have impacted this area of the body. But there was never anything there but a vague anxiety . . . and no healing, over and over and over again.

In that Journey weekend, though, I was guided to open into the infinite wisdom in my own body, which in turn led me deeper. Under its guidance, to my great surprise I went not to my colon, but to my heart. And there I discovered a memory that would certainly never have figured on any trauma list.

I was twelve, spending a lovely Sunday afternoon helping my adored father weed his rose garden. Far beneath the surface, though, in that moment of oneness between us, my soul touched his and knew that he planned to die young. All unconsciously, my loving heart decided in that moment, "If he goes early I have to do that, too."

And so, with every beat of my heart, the trumpets of doomsday resounded through my body—and especially the cell receptors in the colon: "Your days are numbered. There's a sword hanging over your head. You could die at any time. . . ." No wonder my poor gut had given itself a case of ulcers!

In my process, guided still by the infinite body wisdom, the cells that had stored this pain deep in my heart and gut were opened. I poured out the grief and fear, and finally separated my destiny from my father's. I symbolically cut the energetic ties to his soul's path, and reprogrammed my heart to send out to my cells a message of life and love. And from that day in 2003 to this I have not had one moment of the old grinding pain in that area of the body—and the hovering anxiety that had been my unseen companion for so many years is a thing of the past.

Never could I have found the root cause of that condition using the "my mind's-best-guess-plus-the-therapist's-best-guess" method. After all, I spent several fruitless decades trying to do just that! Nor do I have any idea exactly how, after not having worked on it at any conscious level, the anxiety that prevented me from meditating for forty—yes, forty!—years magically left; or how an addiction to reading fiction that had kept me out of my life for over half a century quietly disappeared over the horizon without so much as waving good-bye. And over the years since then, I have found that I do not need to know "exactly how." Under the guidance of the unseen wisdom at my core, the cells know. That is enough.

And even more important, since that weekend I have felt myself, my life, my business, my relationships, picked up and carried along in the currents of a healing intelligence that continues to astound me even as it sustains me in the love and freedom that I am. I have come Home.

Since that time, I have continued to deepen in Journey-work. In going through the Journey Practitioner Program, I have discovered increasingly how to love myself and let God, Life, the Universe, love me—and that then, and only then, can my love truly pour out onto others. And as I have continued to do this deep healing work, over the past few years the ugly Voice has disappeared almost entirely. I have let go of huge truckloads of childhood pain and trauma; and even more important, I have released the anger and resentment I was unconsciously carrying. The Good Little Tin Soldier rarely makes an appearance now. If she does, my wonderful Journey family members are happy to point it out—and even greater wonder of wonders, I'm happy to listen!

I and my partner of twenty-five years, Beth, continue to heal and grow. The Journey has allowed us to clear issues as they arise rather than stowing them away in our cells to cause trouble later. We are both learning to let go of our positions, strategies and manipulations, and just be present with and to each other. And so, in our marriage ceremony five years ago, we made our vows not to each other, but to "that current of Love and Truth which runs through us and all things, and which we choose to call grace." We are under no illusion that this relationship, like the two of us, is anything other than a work in progress, yet we feel the ongoing creation of this work of art is one of the greatest blessings of our lives. Infuriating at times. Heartbreaking at times. Frightening at times. Bewildering at times. And hugely joyful and awe-inspiring and amazing. This co-creation is probably a lifelong task, and it's one I rejoice to dive into over and over and over again, for each time I emerge with a new treasure.

One of the biggest gifts of this healing has been the emergence seven years ago of a true, life-aligned passion in my life: a passion for helping other healers, especially other Journey practitioners. This deep vein of purpose running through my days gives me a sense of zest, excitement and delicious forward movement into the Unknown. As a result, I now have a thriving Journeywork and coaching practice focused on helping other healing practitioners.

A few years ago my personal journey took me beyond healing into leadership. As a self-proclaimed "servant leader," I had always pulled back, pushing others into the limelight, facilitating them and "unselfishly" staying in the shadows. During the Visionary Leadership classes created by Conscious Company (sister organization to The Journey), I realized that I was in fact serving no one by holding back the light and truth that could come through me. Three weeks later, fellow practitioner Joanna Kennedy and I co-founded the North American Journey Practitioners Association. As president, I am delighted to be the visible focal point for our professional development: to hold seminars, to write, to teach, to consult; to serve, yes, and to lead, visibly or invisibly, vocally or silently, as I am led by Life.

Oh, and the Black Cloud? Gone. Permanently, it seems. It's been nine years now—time enough for three of the old cycles—and no Cloud. Just more and more healing, more and more real joy, more and deeper love with my partner, herself now a Journey practitioner, my son and daughter (one a shamanic Journey practitioner, the other a practitioner-coach) and my beloved Journey family.

Do I still experience pain? Yes. Pain, it would seem, is part of the human condition. Suffering, though? I can honestly say, no. Because I've found I no longer have to be identified with my pain—the Truth is always there, even in pain, deeper than the pain, sustaining me no matter what. I choose, almost all the time now, to open into that deeper Truth beneath the pain and to let the pain burn up whatever it needs to. Anything that can burn, anything flammable, is ephemeral, unreal, and when it catches fire, it's ready to go. And in the heart of that healing flame, instead of hurt, there is bliss; instead of the fires of hell, an ocean of Love.

And my story of Journey miracles is not yet finished. For unknown to me, a deeper toll had been taken on my body than I was aware of, and a greater gift lay in store for me than I could have imagined. Here, as I experienced it at the time, is the latest chapter in my healing journey.

It was mid-March of 2009, and I was on staff at one of our Visionary Leadership classes. On the second night I was just drifting off to sleep when I was overcome with a flood of terror unlike any I had ever experienced; I couldn't breathe and felt like there was an elephant sitting on my chest, which was hurting intensely. I wondered if it could be something physically wrong with my heart (I had been a bit out of breath the previous few days) but figured it was just an emotional clearing-out, and after some hours I ended up going to sleep. The following day my chest was still sore and I was out of breath, but it felt more as if my ribs were out. I promised myself I'd get it looked at as soon as possible.

Given both the schedule and my lingering work-till-you-drop attitude, a week went by before I was able to take some time to process this issue. By that time the pain was quite intense, but I was still opting for "ribs out"—until another staff member facilitated me in an inner Journey. There, my primary inner healing guide and mentor got right into my face and literally shouted at me, "Pat, this is not something to ignore. This is a serious wake-up call. You've got some heart muscle damage here; it can heal, but only if you rest for at least six weeks, see these four healers, etc., etc." He gave me specifics as to what to do, who to call, how many Journey processes to do at what intervals.

Having never been spoken to in that fashion by my usually very gentle inner mentor, I went home and followed orders. And sure enough, all four of my healing practitioners (all of whom, as well as their physical healing specialties, use some form of medical intuition or body kinesiology analysis) independently confirmed the same thing. Yes, I did have ribs out, and that had affected the nerves going to the heart and lungs. But that wasn't all. There was more heart tissue damage than that alone would account for. In fact, about a third of the heart tissue was in bad shape, dead or dying.

Knowing that I had inherited two heart defects from my father, I took heed. I rested and processed out a lot of stored grief, especially from the lifelong pattern of recurring heartbreak I was just now beginning to see. I had already released the pain and trauma of many, many individual memories of giving my heart and soul, my love and trust to a person or an organization only to have the recipient punish, reject or betray me. But I had never actually seen before that all these individual incidents were strung together into a story line, a tale of repeated heartbreak that I had adopted as "the story of my life."

Four weeks went by. My health care team had done their

work. I had rested. The ribs were once more in place. Yet I was still having some chest pain. And that elephant was still sitting there, most days.

Easter Monday morning, April 13, I woke gently into that space of pure knowing that comes before the mind kicks in for the day. And in that silent space I quietly knew that this "heart thing" had about an 85 percent chance of carrying me off within five months, and I had better put my affairs in order. It was odd, because there was no emotion attached to this knowledge at all. Nor was there any urge to "do something about it." In fact, the strongest feeling was that, well, death could be a relief, because I was so-o-o tired. Could it be that it was simply time for me to move on to another plane of existence? Was I done? After all, my father died of a heart attack when he was much younger than I am now. I knew I had the same two congenital heart issues, and at age twenty-two had been told I had the heart of a seventy-eight-year-old woman. I had worked hard to keep that heart going over the years, but maybe my time was up.

So I called my dear friend Moe Skaro, who in addition to being an excellent Journey practitioner and body worker is also an amazing medical intuitive. She said, "Well, Pat, as I've been working on you I've had the same feeling that you could be on your way out. So even though it may take four or five weeks to get an appointment, would you be willing to do a session with my teacher, Linda Dean [a well-known medical intuitive]? She may at least be able to help you decide if you want to live or die."

I resigned myself to waiting—and the following morning I had an appointment! We did a deep, deep session in which

Linda asked me what my soul was working on this lifetime. Tuning in, I heard the word "atonement."

Linda: "So what has been the strategy your soul has used in order to atone?"

Pat: "The pattern of heartbreak, over and over, learning from a young age to open up to others who would then reject me . . ."

Linda: "So, ask your soul: is the atonement complete?"

Pat: "Yes."

Linda: "And is there anything left for your soul now?"

Pat: "Well, it could be interesting to see what life is like without this strategy!"

And I began thinking that perhaps there could still be a reason to live . . .

I got off the phone, got into my car and drove an hour to Boulder for a session with Moe. During that session, I asked my inner mentors, "Why do I have this feeling of my life coming to a dead end?" And in answer I received not words but an image.

I saw a railroad line with a smaller branch line running into it at an angle. And I was the Little Engine That Could, running down the branch line, ignoring the red lights that tell the train, "You're coming up to another line, the tracks are switched against you, it isn't safe to go onto that main line yet." So I had come to a crashing halt. I literally could not move on to that other line (going in another direction into a future I could not yet see) until it was safe. And until I had rested and let go of both my heartbreak and my ongoing workaholic pattern, it would not be safe to move ahead.

I saw. And I made a decision for life.

Then I got back in my car and drove back up to Northern Colorado to receive yet another Journey process from a fellow practitioner. And in that session, I told everyone who had ever rejected me, that I got it. I thanked them for being my teachers, for helping my soul by keeping that old pattern in my face until I could see it and let it go. And so I cleared it all out. Forgiven. Done. No longer useful.

So I had processed and processed and processed, three deep processes in a day . . . and in fact I did sleep better that Wednesday night than I had in a long time. And the elephant on my chest was definitely lighter the next day. I had some energy work and bodywork done during the day, and that evening I did a fourth process, in which I cleared some old vows that were keeping me from honoring myself. And that night . . .

That night, instead of the sweet sleep one might think I'm about to report, I had the worst night, physically speaking, of my life. I spent most of it sitting up doing energy work on myself trying to keep my stuttering heart going. Still no panic, just a firm, calm decision: I would like to stay alive here, if possible.

Somewhat to my surprise I made it through the night, and then I called Moe. (I wasn't sharing much of the week's events with my partner, Beth; I just didn't know what to say.) Moe, gently, knowing my "I-have-no-health-insurance-can't-eat-hospital-food-have-paradoxical-reactions-to-almost-all-meds" hospital phobia, told me to talk to Beth and get to the emergency room, and if they wanted to do a procedure,

Moe would come up and be my watchdog, 24/7. "I'm good at getting results," she informed me. As if I didn't know.

I followed orders and went in for five hours of tests: blood work, X-rays, CT scan, EKG, heart monitors. ("We'll give you something for the pain." "No, thank you; I have bad reactions to all pain meds." "Well, we'll find something that will work." "No, thank you; I prefer to know what's going on in my body." Et cetera.) After about four hours, though, the pain was going down on its own, and I could breathe better and better.

Then came the results. "Well," said the very sweet young doctor, "we've tested everything—and your results are textbook perfect! Your heart and lungs look like the heart and lungs of a healthy person less than half your age; your oxygenation is 97 percent (that of a healthy athlete); all your blood values are right in the center, just exactly perfect; your heart rhythm is absolutely steady, just what we want to see. Guess there wasn't anything wrong after all."

Beth and I looked at each other and drew breath to celebrate. And suddenly a huge wave of the blackest self-loathing washed through me, and that nasty-beyond-belief Voice made a dramatic reappearance. It recited all my shortcomings since the age of fifteen and told me what a terrible person I was for upsetting my spouse and my friends like this, there never had been anything wrong with me, it was all just drama, etc., etc., etc.—two hours' worth of filthy "etc." And just when I was beginning to be able to speak again, another wave hit—this time all the beliefs and decisions around "I have to be sick to death in order to rest" that had contributed to the heart issues came flooding up. I sobbed and sobbed and sobbed. I sobbed through the grocery store checkout line. (The doctor had decided it was indigestion and I should take Prilosec.) I sobbed through the rainy drive home. I sat in my armchair and sobbed some more. How could I have done this to myself, to everyone?

Meanwhile, Beth was sitting on the sofa reciting the following mantra: "Call Moe. Call Moe. Call Moe. Moe will know what to do. Call Moe."

"But I'm so ashamed! How could I have done this? How could I have so misread my own knowing? And how could all the others who had independently looked at me and . . ."

"Call Moe. Call Moe. Call Moe . . ."

So when I could finally draw breath again, I called Moe. And Moe said, "First of all, I did see the shadow of death on your heart, Pat. And I saw a lot of dead tissue. And so did Linda. It was undeniable. So now, let's review what happened Wednesday."

Pat: "Wednesday? Well, first I had a process with Linda."

Moe: "And did you see through a major pattern in your life?"

Pat: "Yes."

Moe: "And then what happened?"

Pat: "Well, I did a process with you."

Moe: "And at the end of that session, had you made a deep decision about something?"

Pat: "Yes, I decided to stick around if possible."

Moe: "And then?"

Pat: "Well, I had a process with Sheri."

Moe: "And did you let go of something?"

Pat: "Yes, I let go of that old pattern and forgave myself and everyone else."

Moe: "Well, then, is it possible . . ."

(And even before she says the next words, my body is tingling with the truth . . .)

"Is it possible that you've had a spontaneous healing here? And that that rough night and day happened because the cells had opened and were letting go of the accumulated adrenaline of a lifetime?"

And I saw the perfection of it: first, the physical detox, then the previously hidden self-hatred being released, and finally the underlying beliefs and vows pouring out. And yet, such is our automatic belief in authority at times, I had not even thought to question the doctor's assumption that there had been nothing wrong in the first place!

What I know now is that my body had already spontaneously healed before I even got to the emergency room. The cell memories stored in my heart, the whole long story of heartbreak, had been finally released. No longer needed, the chemical distortions had been expelled into the bloodstream, and I was just experiencing the resulting detox, the aftershocks. And yet through that ER experience, difficult as it was, grace provided me with medical evidence that healing had taken place. I have the X-rays, the blood results, the EKG tape . . . textbook perfect.

And I have much, much more. Since that day—since that very day—I have clear evidence that I am in far better health than I have been in years. Yes, I still need more rest and sleep than I thought I did before, and for a few weeks my body felt as wobbly and nap-prone as if it was recovering from major surgery (as in a sense it was). Yet since then I have been gardening, walking, cycling, running up stairs and down, shoveling snow, working out at the gym without the slightest difficulty. I regularly shovel over a foot of snow off my patio and two sidewalks without even breathing hard, and earlier this year beat a woman twenty years my junior in an informal fast-walking race. My brain is working better than it has in years; I can feel the ample oxygen doing its magic. My chest can expand normally; I have lost pounds of edemic fluid; my appetite is back. I feel energetic and alive!

And there is another miracle there, for me a far more important one. Even after all my Journeywork, I had still had a hard time letting go of my go-for-broke workaholism, my out-of-balance desire to serve, serve, serve at all costs. And though the ugly Voice was much quieter than years ago, it had by no means completely disappeared. Yet miraculously, since Heart Day I am not only healthy, I am truly happy. Lifelong stories and strategies, ongoing patterns of reactivity and triggering, *including that Voice,* are simply gone— without my having to work on them consciously. No more heartbreak: I find myself in love with this world and everyone in it. And my mind is singularly quiet these days. In fact, very often this dyed-in-the-wool workaholic finds herself just sitting for long periods of time, with no thought at all, in pure wonder at the love and light running through this world and through body, heart and soul. I walk through the world at a more gentle pace, enjoying the beauty I have been too busy to see.

Now, almost three years later, new phases of my life have opened up, new and delightfully satisfying avenues of service, and the little engine has moved gently onto the new track, with even more opportunities and actions appearing on the horizon. My life's purpose has expanded in joyful and miraculous ways. And when action is not being called for, I am so happy just to sit quietly resting, waiting in gratitude for Life to move the switch. And loving it all.

Will this life of mine ever be completely pain free, free of all inner burning, all inner fear and terror? I sincerely hope not, for then it wouldn't be life, with all its challenges and uncertainties and lessons and surprises. This current running through my life, this sense of connection with all the Universe, this knowledge of myself and all of us and everything as part of the perfect, ever-shifting design of All That Is—this is the wellspring of joy in my life. And this current I call grace is, above all, movement, change, contrast: ever challenging, ever responding to its own challenge. I love to dance in this design, never knowing what new partners, what new twists and turns, what new intricacies of color and pattern and music will appear next. I may be out of breath at times, I may be whirled in impossible directions, lifted up, cast down, ahead, behind, beside, weaving in and out through galaxies and stars and our own dear and beleaguered planet; I may be out of breath, yes—and mostly it is because I am laughing. Laughing in love at myself in my blindness sometimes; laughing with my fellow singers in the harmony of this creation; laughing for joy.

May we all sing together as the morning stars sang together in joy so long ago, and still do. And may we all laugh together as our healing journeys take us wherever our souls have woven our dance.

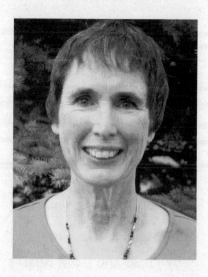

Patricia Kendall *is an Accredited Journey Practitioner, Certified Conscious Coach and Licensed Spiritual Health Coach. Canadian by birth, American by residence, she takes great joy in supporting Journey Practitioners throughout this continent as cofounder and current president of the North American Journey Practitioners' Association. Pat's Journey practice welcomes all who seek healing, with a focus on survivors of childhood abuse; she also loves to assist healers of all kinds. Visit her websites at www.lifepathconsulting.com and www.journey forhealers.com or email her at patkendall@lifepathconsulting.com. Pat shares the beauty of northern Colorado with her partner, Beth, their four cats and her delightful Colorado Journey family.*

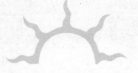

3

Back Issues

by Jared and Ilene Beal

JARED:

In the fall of 2003, I was doing what I do now—excavation, doing heavy lifting—when I came back to Utah from a trip to New Mexico and noticed my back was hurting pretty badly. If I tried to do anything manual, I would be in bed for three or four days, unable to move; the pain was intense. I say "in bed," but actually for three or four months I couldn't lie in bed at all; I had to sit upright on the couch all night. Finally, I tried lying down again, but it took me a month to get to where I could sleep in a bed at all. So I got an MRI and discovered that I had two lumbar discs that were bulging and pinching my sciatic nerves. I tried diet to help me with the pain, and that did take the pain down by about half. But when I'd get out of a car, I would walk like Igor the hunchback . . . bent and leaning to one side. If I went to the grocery store, I'd have to hang on to the grocery cart handle for a long time, bent over like a little old man, till my back would finally loosen up enough for me to walk. Every time I went from sitting to standing, I would feel like an ape-man learning to walk upright, all bent over till . . . ah, now I can be normal! To sit down for dinner was like murder. If I sat down, I never knew how long it would take to stand up. Not great for someone working in construction! Of course, I couldn't lift anything; I could only work the machines. And if I overdid things, even as I tried to regain strength, it would put me back down again. If you'd asked me for the story of my life at that time, I'd probably have said nothing. I didn't like talking to others much anyway, certainly not "sharing my story." But inside I would have heard three words echoing: pain, anger, depression.

Two years later—not a fun two years—my mother-in-law gave us a book called *The Journey*. My wife, Ilene, read it, loved it and said, "Maybe you should read it, Jared." "Yeah, maybe." But I didn't. I had enough on my plate. Then one day that spring I got dragged to our local herb shop to hear an introductory talk for some workshop called the Journey Intensive weekend. Getting ready for boredom, I looked around and saw the presenter, Skip, walking into the herb shop with a woman. As he talked about the Journey-work, something went off inside me. Then Skip turned to the woman he had arrived with. "This is Elizabeth," he said. "She was in a wheelchair for ten years—before she discovered The Journey," and he invited her to share her story. After hearing what Skip and Elizabeth had to say, I knew exactly what I needed to do. I turned to Ilene: "I don't know what *you're* doing, but *I'm* going to that Journey Intensive!"

We both went. I spent my first Journey Intensive half in the chair, half on the floor. It was challenging not to be able to sit upright and to still have to stay alert and listen, but it was well worth it. I felt my buried "stuff" trying to come up, and I'll admit that scared me. When it was time to do our first Journey process, I wanted to run so badly I headed for the door. "What have I got myself into?" But that same woman, Elizabeth, was standing by the door. She said, "This is where you want to be." Looking at her, now standing upright after ten years of sitting in that wheelchair, I agreed to stay and work through whatever was creating such havoc inside of me.

During that weekend what came up, surprisingly, was an old issue with my brother. For twenty years there had been contention between us, and when I wasn't outright fighting with him, I had been silently sending him anger. One time we had been in a really bad fight, and I had ended up walking home, ten miles, fueled by my anger all the way. In the process that weekend I released that anger and came to a place of real forgiveness.

The day after the Journey Intensive, I saw my brother. "C'mere," he said, "I have something for you"—and instead of a kick or a punch, it was a twenty-dollar bill! "Heard you might need this for that trip you're going to take," he added.

I looked at him dumbfounded: "Are you the same brother I grew up with?" The old anger was gone—on both sides. That was when I learned that this Journeywork doesn't just affect the person who does the process. When *you* let go of the old stuff *you're* holding on to, the anger or resentment or hurt, the other person is free to change, too. And as often as not, they do. I've since seen that over and over, at work, in my family, with my friends and relatives. I've changed, and my world has, too.

I first noticed that my back was healing after I let go of that anger; it was looser and not as painful. Little by little, I stopped noticing the pain so much, and by early 2007 the pain was gone. These days I can actually lift more than I could before my back got bad. I've had no relapses, even though I've been lifting pretty heavy stuff. Yet that's only the beginning of the healing that's taken place.

I have also fought a non-physical battle in my life . . . against depression. When I was growing up, boys didn't show emotion, so I didn't either. Now after many more Journeys, I feel comfortable to be exposed in any emotion I feel. When anger comes up, or sadness, sometimes I handle it well, sometimes not so well; but I can embrace the emotions rather than avoid them. Now it's okay if big boys cry!

My relationship with my dad has changed a lot because of that. Instead of being afraid of him and holding resentment and anger toward him because of how I was raised "by hand," I can now love him for who he is. One time recently he came out to my house to spend the day and ended up teaching me welding, a skill he had used all his life but never taught me before. And instead of getting into conflict with him, I was able to see the gift of his knowledge and feel real gratitude, and thank him.

It wasn't just my dad I had been scared of. When I was growing up I was scared of adults, period. I hated to talk to adults—they might yell at me and beat me like my dad did. When I was with my best friend one time as a kid, I accidentally bopped him with a shovel, and his mom came out like a tiger and laid into me, yelling and screaming just like my dad. So I learned, "Yep, adults are scary. It's not safe to be around them." When I "emptied out" with my dad in my inner process one time, I took that old limiting belief and cleared it, and then decided it really was safe to talk to adults. Now I feel comfortable talking to others. I can even talk to more than one or two at a time—I can get up in front of a roomful of people, share my story and speak what's in my heart, and that feels good. If sharing what has happened to me and how I have changed can help even one person who's like I used to be, I want to do that.

The biggest thing is that The Journey has saved my marriage. Now Ilene and I can both take a deep breath when things are triggered and talk it out as we need to instead of just acting and reacting. In the past, for instance, when I would get upset I would just blame Ilene . . . and blame her and blame her. These days I will stop, apologize and say, "Just a minute. I'm broadcasting something here; let me see what's really going on." Then I'll come back to her and say, "This is what was really going on," in a gentler tone, taking responsibility for my own emotional state. As a result, we're a lot more open with each other. And instead of a fight lasting days or weeks, in less than a day we are back to being tender with each other. We have gotten to where we can work through it and forgive, and just be there for each other. Now, if Ilene has something coming up, I've learned to move from, "You just need a process!" to, "I can tell you're going through something. What's here?" Instead of being reactive and playing Mr. Fixit, it's now more like, "Take the time you need to work through this, and when you're ready, let's talk."

My kids can tell the difference, too. My father yelled and spanked us a lot, so another reason for going to the Journey workshops was to break that chain with my own kids. I now have a more tender relationship with my kids: instead of yelling at them, I've learned to say, "So what's going on for you, what happened in your day?" Soft voice: "Let's talk." Now I can really meet them on their level instead of, "I'm the dad, so I'm right." Our second boy, Sam, age eight, now says, "Oh, you're going to another Journey thing? Great! I'm glad you go to those! You come back better." They like being listened to and that we can be open on their level. It's not just, "Dad's the boss," the domineering parent-to-child thing I experienced as a child. It's one-on-one open relating to our kids.

We also use the processes with our kids. When big things come up and we can tell they need the help, we offer a process. My daughter, for instance, was having a big problem with math; we did some Journeywork to find the root cause, resolved it and the issue is gone. Math and my daughter get along fine now.

There have been other things I've needed to let go of, some from early in my life, some very recent. In November 2008, I was working on a job in South Jordan, Utah. I was in charge, and the truck boss named Dave came to help. When he was running the loader, he got out to help another guy, and the loader ran over him. It had pinned him against the curb box and crushed him to death, two days before his fortieth birthday. When the EMTs arrived, I helped pull him out of the hole to put him in the ambulance; he felt like Jell-O, every bone in his body crushed. He had had a brand-new house and everything to live for. That was the worst day of my work life, for sure. I even told Ilene that I never wanted to run equipment again. I was in shock. Then my lovely wife gave me a process called a Phobia Cure, and I was able to go and be there for my boss, and be a support for him through everything that followed. Still, there was a residue: *I* asked for the help, it felt like my fault. Nine months later, my blood pressure soared; I had to take three weeks off work, and I had to do some Journeywork to process the guilt. I did several processes on that—I now realize it was not my fault. I don't have to keep that inside under pressure anymore, so my blood pressure has come down.

At work, they all say now, "Wow, you're the nicest guy I know! You're so calm!" People come and talk to me a lot; they feel the safety, the love, the lack of judgment. They tell me how their day has gone, tell me their stuff, their sorrows. And the next time we meet, there's more of a smile to them. And there's more of a lightness and a smile on *my* face, too.

Construction workers are a rough crowd usually. And if a construction worker like me can tell his experience, they know they can work through things and change their own lives. I love to give back in this way. I've been given a pretty good gift here: recovering from my back condition without surgery and living through high blood pressure. Not to mention the healing in my marriage and my family, and inside of me. Now I have a very positive outlook on life. When there's an issue coming up for me, I know that eventually I'll find a key to it, uncover it, clear the issue, be better, do better. I know in the end, when I look at the issue and clear it, I'll be so much better. I have found more peace in doing Journeywork than I have found in anything else.

Advanced work at the Visionary Leadership courses took the rest of the shyness out of me and helped me go deeper. It allowed me to be more at peace with myself and more in tune with the gifts that I do have. Instead of avoiding different aspects of myself, I can embrace them all and know I am okay. It's like a deep cleaning: a body cleaning, a mind cleaning, the ability to get through your fears, and freedom from guilt and self-punishment. Knowing that I can just welcome it all, that it's all here for a lesson, means I can move forward. It's that confidence that allows me to let myself off the hook and just be okay with who I am.

In the past, it was always everyone else's fault. The big difference is that I don't blame others for my problems anymore. I've gone from, "It's *your* fault" to knowing this is *mine*. I am accountable and responsible, yet I let the situation be what it is. It's an experience: What can I learn from it? How can I grow? What can I get out of it? I've learned to put the blame down; an experience is just an experience, and I'm here to learn.

The Journey gave me back the ability to love myself unconditionally. I grew up under a burden of self-hatred, guilt and judgment. I have learned to let go of the guilt and be who I am, to enjoy it and be happy. I've learned to let go of, to stop owning, society's burdens. Now I know that society's issues don't have to weigh me down. It doesn't matter what anybody says, because it's usually not my stuff anyway. I can relax.

Yes, I'm grateful The Journey helped me to heal my back without surgery and keep the job I love to do. And I'm even more grateful for all the healing I didn't expect: the gift of my wife, my kids and my whole self. I can now feel more of what I want in life and more of who I am. Instead of being a numb zombie going through my day, I have stepped into the aware, alive me—reawakening to my body and being in tune with it. Saying to each new experience, "Oh, this experience—I can learn from it. And wow, feel the happiness that's here with this discovery. I'd like to create more of that in my life!" And there's a lot of joy in that. My world has gone from black and white to Technicolor.

ILENE:

The physical therapist handed Jared a brochure, and I saw the title: *How to Change Your Occupation*. Before we knew it, the therapist had made an appointment for us with a back surgeon and told us that the doctor would be able to get Jared in right away. But that surgery would mark the end of everything we had known, everything my husband had known. He'd always worked in construction! He hadn't gone to college because the job was waiting for him after high school. What would we do? And Jared was only twenty-nine years old! With hardware in his back, I knew our life would drastically change. We had to do something different, and we had to do it now. I didn't sleep that night.

Jared had suffered for eight months by then, and something had to be done; but this felt wrong. "There must be other ways before choosing back surgery," I thought. In the morning, after a long conversation, we decided to call the surgeon and cancel. Good decision, maybe even a narrow escape. We later discovered this particular surgeon had a lot of open space in his schedule for a good reason; his nickname turned out to be "The Butcher."

So I got started with The Journey to fix my husband's back. My mom gave me *The Journey* book that Christmas, and then there was that first Journey Intensive, and Jared's back began to heal. So I put the book, and the work, back on the shelf as we focused on Jared and healing his back. After all, it was his problem, not mine, that we had to solve.

Then in March 2006 we had our fourth child, and I suddenly went into a really deep depression. Everything in my world was falling apart. I was deeply unhappy, I kept fighting with Jared and seemed to have decided that I wanted a divorce. It was very emotional and completely draining. Three months later, I really *was* ready to get a divorce; I believed my life would never get better. All I could think was, "I've gotta get a divorce."

My mom said, "Wait a minute. You've got four kids. Why not give it one last shot and try to fix your marriage before you throw in the towel? There's another Journey Intensive in Colorado next weekend." She volunteered to watch the kids while we both went for my last-chance try.

Being stuck with Jared in the car for the eight-hour drive was good; we had to talk. And that brought up a lot for me.

Then in my Journey process, I discovered that four years previously I had made a vow that if he ever did "this"—an old behavior of his that triggered me—again, I would divorce him. And I realized that right after the birth of our son, that old behavior of his came up again, and *that* had catalyzed the depression I couldn't pull myself out of. That voice in my head was trying to get me to keep to that old vow!

As soon as I found and changed that old limiting vow, the voice that was chanting over and over in my head "I've gotta get a divorce, I've gotta get a divorce" came to an end. I decided that we had four beautiful kids who deserved a healthy mom and dad, and I resolved to be part of making the marriage work. Just that one process shifted my whole attitude and took the pressure off. I was able to sit back and look at the big picture. There was a part of me that loved Jared and my kids and didn't want to throw all that away. That process took away the battle that was going on inside my mind.

On our eight-hour car ride back to Utah, Jared and I agreed to commit to working on our marriage, and I made the decision to trust my husband. We agreed to do more Journey courses and each to work on our own stuff, clearing out the things that were making us turn on each other. And now that my head was clear, I could actually turn my attention to working on *my* stuff. We decided to take some more Journey courses.

After the Manifest Abundance retreat, my greatest intention was to have peace, joy and harmony in my home. And it happened almost instantaneously. It happened first within me, then within Jared, and when we went home, that home was different. It became a safe place; the yelling stopped, and the peace and harmony grew. So we decided to go to The Journey's weeklong No Ego retreat to work even more deeply on our fixated ego patterns.

For us, working in tandem on our personality and ego patterns and taking the seminars together was hugely effective in strengthening our marriage. We'd each have a process and then get together and discuss the things we were learning about ourselves, about our egos and the freedom that was coming. I recognized that I had played the role of victim and martyr in our relationship. "Poor Ilene" could go now. I had a lot of fear and safety issues, too, wanting to know our marriage was safe. When I healed those issues, things could relax. And on the car ride home from No Ego, I first decided to help other families, not just mine. If this could help *my* family so much, it surely could help others find that balance in themselves and in their family life.

I decided I needed to take the final course, Life Transformation—the final week in the Journey Practitioner Program—and Jared wanted to go, too. We asked the kids how they would feel about our being away for over a week, and Sam, our four-and-a-half-year-old son, said, "Yeah, Mom, we want you and Dad to go because you're so much happier after." The other kids echoed that. Our seven-year-old even said, "Yeah, Mom, it's okay. We won't miss you." Our kids were developing real self-confidence on their own!

After we had done Life Transformation Week, though, Sam developed a behavior problem where he was marking the walls with black Magic Marker. My sister, who had also gone through the Practitioner Program, did a Kids' Journey with Sam, and after the process Sam came out of the room and said, "I love you, Mom, and it's okay."

"What's okay?"

"Well, you said I was a bad boy, but now I know you didn't really mean it, and it's okay."

And in that moment I realized I had been saying *he* was bad instead of just talking about the behaviors. Sam went into that process believing he was a bad boy and acting accordingly; he came out knowing "I am a good kid." His behavior shifted hugely from that point on. He *is* a good kid! The direction of his life got altered with one Journey process. And now *I* speak much more consciously. It's a good thing that Journeywork can clear up some of my mistakes, so my kids don't have to carry them forward in their own lives!

Just one vow had nearly ended my marriage; just one belief had affected my son profoundly; and just one changed belief or vow altered life completely for each of us. This began my career as the "Vow Change Queen," changing limiting vows and beliefs stored inside myself and others. I now offer belief and vow changes on a very regular basis as the host of several teleconference calls each month for both practitioners and Journey Intensive "graduates."

Another time my son Hiram stole a small item from a roadside store when we were driving through Arizona on vacation. When he was caught, he was obviously feeling bad about himself and very angry with us for catching him! Jared turned off the radio and said, "Hiram, would you like to do a Journey process?" We did a Journey process right there in the car to help him move through the feelings and figure out his own better way. A few minutes later, he was fine.

When both Hiram's favorite rooster and the cat he had raised were killed on the same day, we buried them both out in the yard and cried till we were done, and then talked about all the good things Hiram had experienced with those animals and how much he loved them. We've learned to let our kids feel what they feel when they feel it, and we have the tools to let them process it through to completion if they need that. We teach them it's okay to feel emotion. If we're sad because the cat dies, we cry about it. And if we need to process something that's sticking, we do. When I backed out of the driveway and ran over a (different) cat, I realized I had a belief that it was my job to take care of everyone, and I was a bad mom because I ran over this four-legged "kid." And just like Sam believing he was a bad boy, my belief that I was a bad mom didn't serve me or the family. So I let that belief go, and I'm a better mom now!

Quite often the processes go beyond my own kids, and they're good with that. When my daughter's friend came to our home and her sister was teasing her about still sucking her thumb in sixth grade, I said, "Hey, I have this cool process that can help with that!"

Michelle just said, "Okay, Mom, you do the Journey process with her and the rest of us will go play outside." Fifteen minutes later, the old habit was gone.

I've also noticed I don't have to overprotect my children anymore. Instead of constantly worrying about whether they'll make it to school safely, I think, "What a great experience they're having going to school!" What a relief, for them and me both!

Journeywork has allowed me to be a better mom and connect with my kids, and to be a better wife and lover to my husband. My life would not be what it is today without The Journey. Today I accept myself and I love myself, and as a result I love and accept everyone around me. I'm not looking for the perfect kids anymore; they can be just as they are. I wake up in the morning and see the light shining through people, the goodness in people. I feel more positive, open and accepting, because behind all the outer blessings lies The Journey's biggest gift to me: the ability to forgive and love myself, and to forgive and love others.

I started out trying to fix my husband and found out I had a few things to fix in myself. Without a doubt, The Journey saved my marriage and my family. By being willing to really look at what I needed to change, I've created a beautiful life: very happy, very secure, very content, and I have so much more to give now than I did before. Then the Visionary Leadership program opened me up even more.

A few years ago I wouldn't have dreamed of giving workshops or speaking in front of others. In the Visionary Leadership program I addressed my fears of failure and discovered what was holding me back from being both the best kind of mom and the best kind of *person* I could be. Now I've found my creative energy, and that's what makes life really fun! I now host many teleconference calls a month, guiding others through group processing and helping our Journey "family" stay connected. I give introductory workshops on cellular healing and Journeywork, and my dream for the future includes creating programs to support families of all kinds through all phases of their development. It's a deep desire of mine to let other people know they can heal their relationships and get in touch with the truth of themselves, their Source, by using The Journey Method.

It was a huge gift for me to be able to present for several months on Vicki Lichtman's Nightly Healing calls, helping folks all across the United States and Canada to take a few minutes together each evening in an intention to connect and heal. We're all very different, yet when we reach out through the heart, we are the same. My life is now directed much more through love, moving from a life filled with fear and protection to a life filled with love, openness and connection. I love to offer this to others.

The greatest lesson? You think it's about forgiving someone else, but it's really about forgiving yourself. Even in that very first process that turned my marriage around, the biggest thing was being willing to forgive myself for my old, unhealthy ways. I did, and my life shifted. I would never have imagined that I would be offering this work, over the phone and in person, to hundreds or thousands of people at a time. The Journey and Visionary Leadership gave me the ability to really tune in inside and speak authentically from my heart to groups of people, regardless of the size of the gathering. Now my vision is to speak to people about families and relationships, to let them know they have the ability to shift and change and create a healthy family if that's what they want. It was what I envisioned those years ago on the trip back from No Ego; and here it is.

I wake up every day now looking forward to the creation in that day, to the life experience it will bring. Helping the world change, one belief at a time, one vow at a time, one cell memory at a time: to me, that is a fulfilling life.

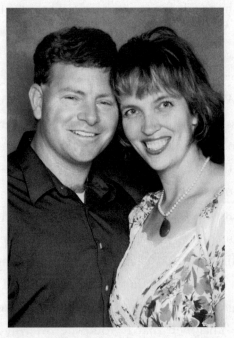

Jared and Ilene Beal *are happily married (fourteen years) and reside in Salem, Utah, with their five children, five cats, twenty-one chickens, and one dog. Jared is running a bulldozer and loader at the local landfill, where he is creating a recycling program. Ilene is a full-time mom. She manages to squeeze in Journey processes and hosts two to three teleconference calls a month. Family comes first these days. Jared and Ilene enjoy planning family activities so they can spend more time together as a family. Their family motto is "The Family That Works Together, Plays Together, Stays Together Forever."*

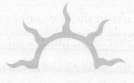

4

Bye Bye Love

by Jasmine Iwaszkiewicz

The bottom had fallen out of my life, and I knew it. I was living a lie. I lived in constant and unprovoked fear and anger: a fear so paralyzing that I could barely bring myself to drive a car, and an anger so vile that my face grimaced with the disdain that I felt for everyone and everything. I loathed my husband, my eldest child asked me to sign guardianship over to his friend's family, and my daughter was a regular at everybody's home but her own.

My life was not what I had envisioned . . . not even close!

My alcohol and drug intake had risen to monumental proportions, my health declining despite my ever-present and committed attempts to exercise, eat well, visit my health care professionals (including the "ist" family of practitioners—the therapists, psychiatrists and psychologists) and lead a holistic life.

Raised in an abusive household with a suicidal mother

and a nonexistent father, survival for me included experiences of homelessness, sexual abuse, streetwalking, gang activity and disease. Lost in the seemingly vast array of human cruelty, I thought I had done quite well: I had managed, for the most part, to avoid feeling the aloneness, abandonment, emptiness and betrayal that plagued my heart.

I began to ask myself, if I had done so "well," then how was it that I was so sick? (I had suffered with severe Crohn's colitis, migraines, asthma, allergies, anxiety attacks, heart palpitations, vein and circulatory disorders and debilitating back, leg and foot pain.) And why was I so unhappy, fearful, violent, angry and blaming?

The answer came in the form of a friend who invited me to attend a Journey Intensive with her. I had no idea of what to expect and had not even read *The Journey*——I was the only one in the room who had not! That weekend changed my life in ways that I had never known to be possible . . .

I walked into the room where the Journey Intensive workshop was taking place and immediately felt embraced and welcomed. The air was filled with the fragrance of kindness, acceptance and love.

Love . . .

That was a new concept for me, to be sure . . .

I can only share this awareness from where I am in my life right now, for at that time, I would have said that I was *the* most open, loving, generous and selfless person I had ever known. This was truth for me, and I had indisputable evidence that this was, in fact, the case. Any time I felt a need to substantiate this perception all I ever had to do was reflect on my past and my present and take stock of how my own mother loved me . . . Or, rather, how she did not love me.

My mother was an addict.

Her drugs of choice were prescription meds: Valium and other wee colorful pills that always seemed to be splayed around our home—when we had one. Occasionally, she would add a heaping measure of alcohol to her recipe for happiness, which created an even more interesting experience of life for me. By the time I was six years old I was quite skillful at being my mother's keeper.

During one of her many unsuccessful suicide attempts, my mother decided that she did not want to die after all. As a result of this momentary choice to live, she told me to dial the telephone operator and tell the emergency dispatcher to send an ambulance. She also instructed me on *exactly* what to say: "Tell them that your mother has just taken too many pills and needs her stomach pumped." In retrospect, I find myself wondering how she was capable of directing her six-year-old daughter to make such a call, in a manner that was coherent and clear, yet she was unwilling to do this herself. It seemed to me that she wanted me to know that she chose not to die. Either that or she wanted very much for me to know that she did in fact want to die—just not on that day . . .

I can still remember my mother telling me that I was a mistake and that she vehemently wished that I was a boy. It became painfully clear to me that I, Jasmine, was not wanted, was unloved and, by all measures, was alone in this world. I knew beyond the shadow of a doubt that if I did not keep my mother safe and alive, then I would die. This was the very simple math of pure survival mode, and over the years I became a gold medalist in the sport of survival.

My mother had left any framework of a balanced type of family life behind when she left my then-believed-to-be "father." This took place on my eighth birthday. My "daddy" was the only frame of reference that made my childhood seem at all normal, as at least his presence conformed to the outer picture of what a family "should" look like.

The man I knew as my daddy was also an addict. His "drug" of choice was gambling . . . I remember that he would stay out for days, and my mother would worry and tell me that *if* he hit it big, then we would celebrate. This happened a lot—the celebration part—or maybe it just seemed that way . . . because those celebrations are some of the only happy or love-filled memories that I have of my childhood, and in particular, with a man.

My daddy came home one day after a very long gambling streak, and when he walked in the door, I could tell that things were not quite right anymore. It is amazing what we know when we are children. And, for me, being a child meant that I had no control over any outcome, choice or decision. I was simply along for the ride—an unwanted passenger on what felt like the "crazy train."

My daddy's face was ashen and wildly unshaven. His always beautifully groomed clothes were wrinkled and disheveled, his fragrant scent foul. What drew my attention the most were Daddy's eyes. There were dark circles under them, and they seemed hollow and old. It was as though he had aged one hundred years before my very scared seven-year-old eyes.

I watched as my mother looked at him, and I knew from her reaction that I was correct in my young conclusion; something was very wrong. That was when the screaming began. My mother was livid, and as she threw words of hate and violence toward my daddy, all I could feel was sorry for him.

He skulked off into the bedroom that he shared with my mother and took a long shower. Afraid to move, I remember sitting very quietly in the living room as my mother somehow became calm, as though nothing had happened, and began to prepare dinner. I found myself comforted by this—the familiar smells of her cooking and the hot rising scented shower steam that found its way into the living room where I sat on the couch.

I felt a welcome wave of relief float through my body as my daddy entered the living room and sat beside me on the couch. I noticed that my mother was strained, and I was afraid, so I did what I had learned how to do best—I decided to distract everyone from what was happening by luring their attention away from themselves and their volatile emotions. This was a skill that came from feeling responsible for controlling and directing my mother's emotions. I knew with every fiber of my being that my life depended on being the "emotional barometer and adjuster" in my household—and everywhere else.

In other words, I was hyper-aware not only of my mother's ever-changing emotional state but of everyone else's, as well. I had developed some kind of unique and unparalleled version of what I now refer to as my "Spidey" sense. When this superpower alerted me to even the subtlest of nuances of shift in a person's state, at the speed of light I could (and still can) *know* exactly what they were feeling, and how they were about to act. If their impending emotions felt in the slightest of ways dangerous, I would distract them or do something for them. This dance of response in relation to others' vibes has served me well in many ways. It also left me feeling totally victimized by and responsible for the whole world—a world that I knew somehow loathed me and was completely unsafe.

As Daddy sat on the couch I noticed, out of the corner of my eye, my new red toy telephone. I skipped over to its place on the floor, picked it up and pretended that it rang. I said, "Hello" and then promptly handed the phone to my daddy and told him that the call was for him.

He looked haggard as he took the receiver and played along with me. I laughed and played the part of what my mother referred to as the "coquette." I laughed and saw that the corner of his mouth lifted up into the beginnings of a smile. This small facial movement spurred me on and I rang the telephone again. This time as I handed it to my daddy he glared at me and said, "Please, Jesse [he always called me Jesse], no more after this, okay?" I looked at him as my mother sat down beside him, smiled and told him to play with me because I had missed him while he was away. She was right, I had. Spurred forward by my mother's act of unsolicited support, I let the phone "ring" and once again handed it to my daddy. Reluctantly and sternly he told me that this was the last time. He explained that he was tired and needed to be quiet. In that moment all I saw was that my family was together, and for once in my young life my mother was on my side and was actually enjoying me. This was all I needed to propel me into an "out of control" state and as a result, I lost all sense of my über-super survival power. I made a mistake. Just one.

This single moment of loss of control on my part taught me very well to never ever allow that to happen again, for in the next nanosecond I quite literally watched myself hand my daddy the telephone for the last time. As my small hand placed the receiver next to his ear, all I saw was a flash of red as my prized toy was hurled through the air at the wall across the room. This broke my telephone, but worse, it shattered my love, trust and belief in my daddy.

In that moment I got it that my daddy no longer loved me, and that he, too, like my mother, was unsafe.

Case closed. Heart closed. Trust shattered. Love destroyed.

In that instant something deep inside of me shut down, and it stayed buried, under lock and key, for the better part of three decades.

The look on Mother's face was extraordinary. And as I cried, I also felt that even though she was attempting to soothe me, it no longer mattered. Cold, icy and stony, I was no longer the same little girl I had been mere seconds before.

Love . . .

The next time I saw Daddy it was a week later. It was my eighth birthday, and I was perched atop a packed box in the middle of the living room. My mother was moving us out and away from my daddy who, as she said, "could no longer be trusted." I already knew that. So, as I sat on that box, I floated above my body. I watched from above as the men helped move the boxes out into the apartment building hallway and into the elevator. I felt as though I was dreaming as I watched Daddy come into the apartment and kneel down beside me. In his hand was a package of pink coconut cupcakes bought from the local grocery store. He looked up at me and tears were streaming down his face as he said to me, "Jesse, I'm sorry I don't have any money, and this is all I could get you for your birthday." I watched my daddy cry with not one iota of feeling toward him. In my mind, he had betrayed me and had destroyed my world, and now *he* wanted *me* to soothe *him*. And so I did. This was, after all, my job. I looked at him from someplace that was far away and almost scientifically detached in nature. I watched him as though he were an experiment, and I spoke the words, "It's okay, Daddy, I understand." And I did. I understood far more than they, or I myself, gave me credit for. I knew that I was alone, and no matter what I did or did not do, the only one I could rely on was myself. And so it was. I lived in a shell of observational isolation, and a team of wild horses would not be able to draw me out. End of story.

I did see my daddy one more time after my birthday. He came to visit me and took me to the corner gas station to fill the tires on my new bicycle. He had bought this new toy for me in an attempt to salve my aching heart and show me that I was somehow all grown up now, and that this new life was so much better than the old one because I was now able to be free: I lived in a house rather than an apartment and had learned to ride a bike. I knew differently. On the inside, I was anything but free—that basic gift of love and trust that comes with life had been stolen from me and it was never coming back. As my daddy walked away from me at the gas station, he promised that he would come back to visit with me the following week, and I *knew* that he was lying. My Spidey sense was new and improved since its small lapse . . . and it was sharper than ever!

I was right. He never did come back.

If I had at that time the tiniest sense of trust or faith left hidden somewhere deep inside of me, it no longer existed after the week had passed, and I never spoke of my daddy to anyone ever again. Not even to my partner and husband of twenty years. That part of my life was off limits and had never existed as far as I was concerned. And quite frankly, I could not have cared less . . .

The next few decades are another story unto themselves. I chose to never get married, never have children and never open my heart.

Interestingly, I did all three.

Truth be told, I opened my heart as far as I could, and somehow it was never enough. I always felt that I had to protect myself from some unseen hammer that was going to drop out of the sky and destroy my life, or worse yet, further break my already shattered heart.

And yet now, walking into this seminar room . . .

Love . . .

Yes, that room was filled with love. IT was everywhere. IT oozed from the eyes of the Journey trainers, the facilitator, the staff, the music, the video, the participants, the floors, the walls, the chairs and the very air. I could not escape and instead found myself beginning to soften—and this scared me to no end.

As the initial teachings finished, the time came when we, the participants, were to buddy up with a partner and try a Journey process with each other while the trainers and staff watched over us like shepherds over their flock. I was excited and found myself chomping at the bit, knowing that I could certainly deliver a process with ease. I was, after all, extremely adept at caretaking and as smart as a whip. This would be easy . . . and it was.

My partner had a simple and apparently powerful experience and I felt that I had done my job rather well. And then it was my turn to receive . . .

As instructed by my partner, I closed my eyes and took a deep cleansing breath, and we began. What I discovered after that changed my life and world forever.

Deep inside my body was where I ventured to—and this is key. For this, this that set me free, was nowhere to be found in my mind, could not be explained by my mind and, cleverly, had been long forgotten by this brilliant mind. And the memory that crept into my awareness with the power of this simple process opened the door to my freedom—a freedom that to this day remains, albeit even vaster than I could ever have dreamed or desired.

I saw my daddy. I felt his presence. I saw myself at the birthday of my shutdown to love, in the scene that I had lived and experienced decades before. I was sitting atop those packed boxes, and I saw the pink cupcakes and his tears. I felt his painful pleading and witnessed my own cold, austere, young, calculated removal of myself.

As I was guided to speak to him, the words that came shook me from within. I shared with him that my pain was never about his leaving my mother. I told him that I understood his leaving, and I did; for if *I* could have left, I would have. It was not about his penchant for gambling or his throwing my telephone and breaking it. This pain was not about the fact that he had no money and could not provide me with a birthday gift. As I spoke with him from this hurt—this hurt that I had shoved deep down into my body in an attempt to not feel the truth and power of it—I realized what this deep and abiding ache was really about.

This hurt—the greatest pain that I had ever felt—was about the fact that he had left *me* behind.

He had left me. He had abandoned me. He had fed me to the hungry and insatiable monster of a woman whom I called Mommy. He had been the cause of all of the subsequent pain, humiliation, homelessness, streetwalking, abuse and suffering that I had ever experienced. It was because of his unwillingness to love me and care for me that I had suffered. It was because of this pain that I had never been able to fully open my heart to and love another . . . especially a man. In that moment of pure clarity and personal inner awareness I saw, felt, heard and knew beyond the shadow of a doubt the ramifications of this pain that I had carried.

I watched the truth, or rather, the falsities, of my entire life unfold before my eyes. I saw how I had shut down to fully giving and receiving love. I was humbled, distraught, forgiven and free. As I sat amid my own tears of clarity, truth and resolution, I offered all that I had to give—I offered my forgiveness. As my heart opened for the first time since I was eight years old, it radiated its song of love. My heart forgave my daddy.

It was in that brief window of a moment in time that I was set free.

When I opened my eyes, I knew by the way I experienced that which surrounded me that I had changed. I had just been transformed. My life was new. It was fresh. My body felt different, lighter somehow. It was as though this body was alive for the first time, and it felt good. My mind was still and content; akin to a small child sucking on a lollipop, it was simply fully entranced and enamored with what was going on in that moment. My mind was, for once, quiet. It was not thinking about what was next or what happened before or what it wanted for dinner or where and how that would take place. It had no worry about my children, my then husband, or my home. It was silent and happy. This was so spectacular that I cried tears of joy and appreciation for what I felt in my body, mind and spirit.

I felt *love* . . . real, unabashed, open, clear, beautiful, juicy, succulent, delicious, joyous, playful, expansive, all-encompassing love.

The most beautiful thing about love is that it grows. Love expands. It is always in motion, and the direction it takes is like a lush, open, floriferous, expansive field of all that is, and it contains all possibilities. This love has no doubt, judgment, blame, story, past or future. This love does not seek, need, want or think. This love is what has carried me forward through my life since that first Journey weekend. This love is what has created my life, and it continues to guide me through the space of my heart. This love tells me what is in integrity for me. This love respects, honors, values and supports. I have come to know that, in fact, I *am* this love. It moves through me. It speaks through me. It shines through me. It *is* me. This love has healed my body, mind, emotions and spirit. It is this love that allows me to assist others in coming home to their own hearts—to be free.

Many years have passed since that first Journey Intensive weekend. I continued along in their program offerings and became an Accredited Journey Practitioner, among other things. The one pivotal scene that I have shared with you from my vast stream of life experiences was the single most profound turn of events that I had known until that time. It was—The Journey was—the tap that finally let flow my own personal inner freedom. And for that I am forever grateful. I honor The Journey and its work from all of my heart and self.

When I arrived home after that first weekend, I shared with my husband what had taken place. As I spoke, his mouth hung open and his eyes stared at me with amazement and awe. He, the man who had known me for twenty years, had been married to me for fourteen years, had watched me birth our two beautiful children, had never ever heard about my daddy, let alone about what had happened. You see, I told my husband that I had no father, and I did not . . . for until that process, my daddy was dead to me, as was my love.

I shared with my husband how I had set up my entire life, and every relationship that I had taken part in, including our marriage, from a place of fear of abandonment and betrayal. I explained to him that I had always been afraid to let him in because until then I "knew" that he would leave me.

I sat on our bed as I shared this with him, and my tears flowed like a river of healed truth and vulnerability. I had opened myself to my husband for the first time and I asked for his forgiveness. I had never felt so naked, so exposed, and it felt like I was standing in the presence of life itself.

My husband is a beautiful man, and he offered me his forgiveness, love and support as I continued along my own path of personal self-discovery, awareness and healing. He stood by me during the times that were challenging, and I honor his role in my life. He has been one of my best teachers and remains a dear and adored friend.

My marriage, though, formally ended a short year and a half after that first Journey weekend.

Truth be told, my marriage had actually ended ten years earlier. And through the Journeywork that I was doing, and my husband's attempt to understand what was taking place as we were both caught up in an ever-shifting swirl of change, we were finally able to say good-bye.

He attended a Journey Intensive and found the truth in his own heart, and he shared that with me three months

later. He told me that he loved me, but he was no longer
in love with me. As those words echoed through my body,
mind and heart, I stood wide-eyed in his presence. I was
dumbfounded. The world stood still on that hot summer
afternoon as we strolled through our garden. He looked
deeply into my eyes and he asked me if *I* was still in love
with *him* . . .

I can remember standing barefoot on the warm summer grass, deafened by his question as I begged for the
right words to come out of my mouth. Nothing came. Not
a sound. The silence was palpable as I searched for the response I thought was true. I thought that I was in love with
my husband, and as I desperately searched for these words
inside, they were not there. All that I heard was my own
heart beating and its song of truth. He was right. I was no
longer in love with him. I, too, loved him deeply and still
do, as a friend—a best friend, as the father of our children,
as a man, as a confidant, as a housemate, as a business partner. I strove to find the *in love* feeling for that man. I dug
deep, and all that I came up with was silence. And in that
clarity of wordlessness we were both set free. The secret
had dissolved . . .

I moved out of our marital home four months after our
last garden stroll. And I want to be crystal clear in this sharing: separating from my twenty-year marriage and partner-
ship was challenging in many ways. It was painful, truthful,
honest, real, open, raw, tender and angry. I cried every day
for six months as my old layers of consciousness, memories,
beliefs, vows and experiences were shed during the year

and a half that it took me to fully heal and begin my life
anew.

I would not trade one moment of that time for anything
in this world. It was through this housecleaning of me that I
grew wings and began to take flight from my heart.

I have shared the story of the ending of my marriage with
many, for one reason and one reason only. I still, to this day,
am in awestruck compassion for the way in which my husband and I moved through this ending and into a new beginning.

We have yet to consult a lawyer. We did not go to court.
We did not fight or argue about custody of our children. We
fairly and honestly decided on the settlement of the marital
assets. We have shared every holiday dinner together since
that warm December day, six years ago, when I left. My
then husband even helped me move and assembled my new
furniture for me. We shared from our truth and hearts with
our children and rode the waves of their pain, as well as our
own, with grace, elegance, sincerity, compassion, nurturing
and love—vast, enormous, epic love.

When I tell this story of how simple, honoring, respect-
ful and full of integrity this all was, people tend to be
amazed—awestruck even. They ask how this can be so. I always respond in the same way: "If we came together in love,
then how is it that we would not separate in love?"

For me, the greatest gift that came from all of this was
the presence of love. As I reflect, I see clearly how we both,
through our mutual honoring and respect of each other and
ourselves, taught our children the truth of love. Real love.

Love that abides no matter what is happening in the outside world. No matter what is taking place, it can all be navigated from a place of love. We, *together*, taught our children about love. We showed them and ourselves that even if love changes its form of expression, it still remains and can in fact grow even deeper and become more expansive and all-inclusive.

We harbor no blame, no judgment, no story, no expectations, no war, no anger, no fear, no gossip, no drama, no abandonment and no betrayal. Even though, if the whole story with all of its glorious details were fully shared, others might wonder in fascination how this could be possible, all I can ever say is, "It is." When we make choices born of love and the truth of our own hearts, our words and actions take on a life of their own and that life, that breath, is governed by peace.

It is for this that I am forever grateful to The Journey. It is because of this that I share with you in this small offering of my simple words, the truth of what *is* possible—endlessly possible . . . vastly possible . . . The only impossibility resides in the mind and in our thoughts of who or what we believe we are "supposed" or " not supposed" to be, say, think, feel or do.

My life today is a shining, brilliant, radiant and love-filled reflection of my heart—of my love, of me. It is unique, fascinating, beautiful, open, clear and resolved. I live in truth, filled with gentleness, kindness, compassion, health, glow and the playful innocence of a child. I live in a state of wonder and amazement for all that is. I am happy, joyful and radiant. I am finally living the life of my dreams. Truth be told, this life that I am living is far more interesting and blissful than I could ever have dreamed possible. Such is the power of Love.

Life IS beautiful. Life IS Love, and Love IS Life.

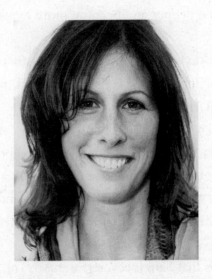

Jasmine Iwaszkiewicz is a practicing Accredited Journey Practitioner, Intuitive Energy Medicine Practitioner, Life Guide, Facilitator, Teacher and Healer who offers one-on-one sessions in person and via telephone. Jasmine facilitates workshops on Relationships and LIFE: Love, Integrity, Freedom & Empowerment. Contact her at Jasmine@ TheAcademyofLife.com.

5

An End to War

by Joseph Doyle

When and where does my journey commence? What was the first step? Who knows? Not I. I only know that many journeys were traveled, the ancestral preludes to mine, and their steps are recorded in my DNA.

I come from a long line of warriors dating back to the time of the Vikings (which literally means "raiders") who ruthlessly invaded, pillaged and fought the fierce Celtic warriors in what has become Ireland. These forebears of mine were berserkers, frenzied fighting machines consumed with bloodlust; and forty strife-filled generations later my own grandfather carried on our family legacy fighting in the rebellion against the thousand-year British rule.

It was the 1920s, and Ireland was experiencing "the Troubles," a period of civil war. My grandfather and his neighbor who had been so active in the rebellion now immersed themselves in the challenge of forming a new government.

They became targets of the opposition, and a grenade thrown into the backyard of the neighbor's home killed the neighbor's son. My grandmother informed my grandfather, "When adults fight, children die. That's enough, you're next, and we're leaving, now." Thirty days later, they were in New York City; Dad was seven years old.

My mother, also Irish, also descended from a long line of warriors and rebels, arrived on these shores as a baby. For both my parents, journeys begun in Ireland ended up in the Bronx. This son and daughter of warrior families met, a new family emerged, and my own personal journey began, as I became the next bearer of this cellular soup of war and strife.

Conceived in war, the Second World War, I was Mom's first pregnancy. During that time her brother Billy and my father's brother, Bobby, were both killed in action. Neither body was ever recovered. War had come to Mom, flooding her with grief. It overflowed into me, and even there in the womb, it seems the vow began—the vow not to feel it, not ever.

I was born by the blade, sliced out in a Caesarian section. Arriving jaundiced, I was isolated from my mother. Mom's hospital stay ended, but I was left, alone in the incubator. It took ten days for the jaundice to clear. Mom, a cardiac patient, was too weak to care for me, so I went to Grandma's. Here, Grandma, two aunts and especially Dad became the primary caregivers. I was showered with attention, constant and loving—just not from Mom. Six months later, Mom, Dad and I eventually got to our own home. But Mom's condition meant that Dad continued as primary caregiver for a few more months. Maternal disconnect was complete.

Somewhere in there, I stopped crying. My aunts tell me I was a "good baby," only crying for food or to be changed, never for attention.

Mom had her war, and it wasn't limited to the one being waged across the seas in Europe and Asia. She had at least six pregnancies, and I was the only live birth. Three brothers were stillborn, and there were at least two miscarriages. I had survived, my brothers had not, and sadness was omnipresent.

Dad had his war, too. As a New York City fireman, he had an exemption from military service due to having a critical occupation. Yet he felt shame: his siblings and in-laws were doing their utmost to defeat Hitler and his allies. They were true heroes. One from each family had already been lost. Dad contrived to get his exemption changed and, joining the navy, left so he could play his part in the war.

Cut from Mom, abandoned by her in the hospital, cared for by others, young Joe had another betrayal. Dad, the caregiver, had departed; the abandonment was complete.

With this second desertion, my sense of having parental approval and love departed. I can't recall making a conscious vow at this time, yet I do know that I have been fiercely loyal all of my life, carrying the conviction that I will *never leave anyone behind*. And just a few short years later, this "vow" was waiting in the wings. It would become the foundation on which I would construct my life.

Mom lost a second brother before the war ended, but Dad returned home safe. Pregnancies began again, and, although I recall only two, my aunt said that it seemed like Mom always had a baby on the way, yet none arrived. Finally, the doctors told her, "Church or no Church, you will kill yourself with another pregnancy," and the pregnancies ended.

We lived in a housing project in the Bronx. It wasn't a city ghetto, but a really nice neighborhood to grow up in. Yet these were the streets of a rough city, where one needed to be tough just to survive.

About the time that I turned ten, I got beat up by two kids. I went upstairs to get Dad, my all-time hero, the man who fought the fire dragon every day and won, to come down and help me. Dad asked if I had fought back, and my tearful "no" brought the most unexpected response: I would have to go back downstairs and stand up for myself, he couldn't fight my battles for me. I remember going back down, thinking that he didn't love me and that I was a coward. So on the way, I made The Vow: I swore to myself, "I will never, ever back down from anyone or anything, as long as I live." From this moment forward peace was lost, and a little boy went to war.

I never shed a tear.

Vietnam was still years away, so street fights and football served instead. Later, bars would replace the street as combat zones, brawls being the most available Viking berserker outlet. Eventually, the United States Marine Corps would become my training ground. Here, the Bronx street fighter, the Viking berserker, the Celtic warrior merged with the finest combat training on earth: a loose cannon became a finely tuned and formidable weapon, one that would be forged into steel by the fires of war.

"Dad, this going to war, this extreme path of life or death, this is how far I will travel to get your love and approval."

The United States Marine Corps, testosterone heaven, the finest fighting force in the universe, the alpha of alpha organizations. It may not have been paradise on earth, but it was *my* Garden of Eden. Grandpa Viking and Grandma Celt had provided the right DNA combo for me to merge into this warrior society. The Marine Corps did the rest.

The Marine Corps has an unofficial motto, at least it did when I served: "A small war is better than no war at all." That resonated in every cell of my being. Every day was preparation for war. I remember in boot camp, the first training stage for recruits, one of our drill instructors had done a couple of tours in Vietnam as an advisor, combat troops not being officially deployed until March 1965. His comment to us "boots" was, "You can't understand combat until you experience it, and none of you have; except maybe Doyle and Sams." (I was a Bronx street product. Sams was from Detroit.)

Training completed, after boot camp we were fine-tuned in the infantry training regiment and assigned to our permanent units. Vietnam was paramount in our thoughts, and on March 8, 1965, the 9th Marine Regiment landed in Vietnam and was assigned the task of guarding the air force base in Da Nang, RVN, from mortar and rocket attacks, snipers and infiltrators. This role quickly expanded from being a reaction force to actively seeking the Vietcong in their hiding places, and combat escalated; eventually it would involve the North Vietnamese Army, too.

I am not going to detail what service during Vietnam was like; I never have shared that, and I don't intend to start now. There have been myriad books and articles penned, where individual recollections can be read. Suffice it to say that the men in my original unit suffered horrendous casualties, many doing second and even third tours. Most of them are now immortalized, their names inscribed on the Wall for all eternity. And there came a point in time that my soul said to me, "Fuck this shit! I'm outta here; you are on your own!"

Vietnam had an effect on my life that is impossible to calculate. It was a constant companion, and I fought it internally every day for more than four decades. I shut down to all the humanity, emotions and love that were showered on me by the Divine. I lived in hatred and rage, tension and conflict, fear and guilt, denying love, happiness, companionship and my right to have them.

I never shed a tear.

I had armored myself in the womb. I felt the sadness that was in my family, and *I* wasn't going to feel that, not ever. I just did not allow myself to feel loss. Of course, I didn't really feel anything else, either. At least not on a conscious level; everything got pushed down. One cannot selectively suppress one emotion. Depress one, depress all. Maybe that is why it is called depression.

I protected myself. I went numb. I did not perceive my enemies as having humanity. They were objects to be disposed of, wiped away, so that I and my brothers in arms could survive. My soul became bleak and desolate. I had no way to nurture it, so I would flood it with alcohol. Just like a flood in nature, the aftermath was even more devastation and wreckage.

I never did transition to civilian life. I took off the visible uniform and gear, but I left every bit of armor in place, enhanced with sword and shield, ready to assail all those who I disliked. Worse, ready to assail those I loved, no matter the cost.

I was still in the Marine Corps when I married Mary-Ellen Sheridan. We met when I was sixteen, she was fourteen—my first love, and I was unaware that I had just met my first Guardian Angel. We dated occasionally, a romance blossomed and we married.

It was 1968, and my job was to turn recruits into combat troops, a total immersion in warrior testosterone. I can't imagine what it took for MaryEllen to stay in the marriage. But stay she did, and in so doing she saved my life.

Alfred, Lord Tennyson honored the victims of one of the great military blunders in history with his immortal poem "The Charge of the Light Brigade." Six hundred men were ordered to charge into a valley, while the enemy occupied the ground and had every inch of turf covered with cannons. It was a death trap, and few survived. Tragedy ruled the day, fueled by the stupidity and ineptitude of the commanding officers. Yet none could question the courage of those who charged.

> *Theirs not to make reply,*
> *Theirs not to reason why,*
> *Theirs but to do and die:*
> *Into the valley of Death*
> *Rode the six hundred.*

> *Storm'd at with shot and shell,*
> *While horse and hero fell,*
> *They that had fought so well*
> *Came thro' the jaws of Death,*
> *Back from the mouth of Hell,*
> *All that was left of them,*
> *Left of six hundred.*

In many ways, this was Vietnam in a nutshell. Sent into a ground war in Asia by inept politicians more worried about careers than casualties, we weren't allowed to reason why, just to do and die.

And when we thought we had come back from "the mouth of Hell," and came home to "the World," we were greeted by hatred and condemnation. I looked at this landscape that I defended at the risk of my life and saw that I was a stranger in a strange land. I had more in common with the Vietcong and the North Vietnamese Army. They were Vietnam vets, too, just shooting in a different direction. We teenagers had served in the belief that we were protectors of our land and its citizens and their right to freedom—and we were vulnerable to the self-serving political hypocrisy of our government.

I became consumed by guilt for having survived. I tried myself for having lived when my brothers-in-arms died. The verdict—Guilty! The sentence—Death! The method—Lethal Ingestion! The toxin—Alcohol! MaryEllen commuted that sentence; she would not enable its execution, and instead I ended up living shackled in the unbreakable chains of my own self-created prison.

I never shed a tear.

MaryEllen began her domestication of the Viking, and her Celtic devotion to the Roman Church brought great dividends: first a son, Brian, then a daughter, Noreen.

Noreen was mine, at least as much as any man can have a baby. She spent most of her short life in a special neonatal care unit in New York City, and I was able to visit her daily. I fed her, changed her and suctioned the mucus from her lungs. She came home for a brief visit, and her heart and breathing stopped. I did CPR on her all the way back to the hospital. She stayed on another month, and then it was her time to depart, and she died.

I never shed a tear.

Mom was next, just a few months later. Her fourth heart operation had a glitch, and she experienced a small stroke.

When sent to a rehabilitation facility, she tried to get out of her wheelchair unaided, fell and fractured her skull. Within a span of twenty days, she underwent open-heart surgery and brain surgery. Her body survived another four and a half years, but I never again had a conversation with my mother. I could only speak *to* her, not *with* her.

I never shed a tear.

In the order of life, normally daughter follows mother. That had not happened. Our life together continued: two more sons arrived, Kevin and Patrick. And then, something uninvited. MaryEllen, always a model of health, found a lump in her breast. A mastectomy ensued, a three-year period of remission, then an eighteen-month trip to oblivion. Mother had followed daughter into death.

I never shed a tear.

Dad was next. I buried MaryEllen at Christmas 1993, and a month later I placed Dad in a hospice. It took six months, and during this time he told me how proud he was of me, and how I had turned out great. But a little boy who went to war to find love and approval could not hear the words or accept the gift. The dying was a rerun of a familiar show, just with a new cast member. My all-time hero died, and I buried him. I was now the sole survivor of that little family begun in the Bronx so many years earlier. Two parents and five unmet siblings were gone. I did not realize it at that time, but the bond that truly held us together was death.

This was the lowest point of my life. Dad and MaryEllen gone, no one to turn to. Totally alone, I was responsible to be both mom and dad for three young boys, and I had no idea how to do that. I wasn't even a good father. How would I ever be a good mother?

Being left alone, not knowing what to do, I resorted to the one tactic that had seemingly worked after Vietnam. After another speedy trial for my failure to be fully emotionally present for Noreen, Mom, MaryEllen and Dad, I came to the same verdict—Guilty! Another sentence passed—Death! The proven method—Lethal Ingestion! Again, the toxin—Alcohol! And no one could stop me.

Not being aware that I had already met one Guardian Angel, I was totally clueless that another one had entered my life. Nancy Mae Alfrey seemed to appear out of nowhere. I know her history now, but at that time it was just wondrous. If she hadn't arrived, I would have in all likelihood drunk myself to death. For the first time in a long time I started actually looking forward to the clock moving forward, instead of trying to wind it back. Death sentence commuted again! Only this time there would be a totally different path to tread, although it would take me a few years to find it.

Nancy came to work for me as my children's nanny, and even though I'm fond of joking that she married me because she liked the title Head of Household much better, the real truth was, she enabled *me* to become the head of household, because there was now actually a household to be head of. That household's foundation is her heart, and on it she built love, connection and understanding.

Yet our connection was not complete. The marriage vow between MaryEllen and me had a life of its own, even though it had been lived to its fullest: "I will love you and honor you as long as we both shall live." There was no longer a "both" for MaryEllen and me; she had left this world, yet I felt guilt that in marrying Nancy, I was cheating on MaryEllen.

Although I was not conscious of this, in truth, I had been twice blessed with Guardian Angels: MaryEllen, who would not allow me to execute my self-imposed death sentence as a failed warrior; and Nancy, who would not allow me to execute my self-imposed death sentence as a failed protector of family.

Nancy understood that there was more to living than this and began her active search to find that. I had had my life saved twice, once by each Angel. For Nancy, that was not enough, there was work still to be done. It was now time to save my soul.

Her search found The Journey.

I cannot say that The Journey has *given* me anything. And yet, at my very first Journey Intensive, in March 2005, I uncovered the vow I had made as a little boy, "I will never, ever back down from anyone or anything, as long as I live"—I unearthed the moment when my last chance for peace was lost, and from then on, a little boy went to war. Yet this time, in my Journey process, I experienced my father's pain at having to make a decision to allow his son to grow, to become his own person. I felt my father's pain at not defending his son from harm, his pain at letting life take his son away.

And, for the first time, I wept.

There was a side benefit, a physical one. At the time of that first Journey process, I suffered from diverticulitis, a condition that led to frequent infections in my colon and necessitated that I carry two prescriptions for antibiotics on my person at all times. The attacks, which came eight to ten weeks apart, could quickly become life threatening if treatment wasn't started immediately. By eight months after that Journey Intensive weekend, not only had I not had an attack, I had actually thrown the prescriptions away. A genuine benefit, and yet that was not the real healing.

At another Journey Intensive a year later, while listening to the story of a man whose eyesight had improved tremendously, I was hit with a further realization. I had heard the story several times, as it is part of the film of Brandon Bays shown at Journey Intensives. In it, the man, named Brian, keeps repeating, "You don't understand! You don't understand!" as he tries to explain how one process healed him.

That phrase, "You don't understand!" kept nagging at me, and I didn't understand why. And then something whispered in my head, "When was the last time you had a flashback to Vietnam?" and I answered, "March 2005." It had been almost two years since I'd had an occurrence of those debilitating flashbacks.

And I wept again.

The Journey has *"given"* me nothing. Yet when I was wracked with the grief of my own war, Vietnam, and the secret grief for my brother Marines that I'd not allowed myself to feel before, I underwent a Journey process supported by a magnificent Journey Practitioner. She was a beautiful feminine soul who enfolded me in an embrace of such sacred maternal love that I can still feel her support today. The son in me felt suffused with love, felt a bond with the Eternal Mother, and I knew my mother's grief for her brothers.

And I wept.

The Journey has *"given"* me nothing. Yet on a day that I was filled with anger and rage, a day that I was ready to do battle, I received a Journey process. In this process, my platoon showed up, as they often did in my processes, and I remember thinking, "What are you doing here? We are finished, you have been honored, and forgiveness has been given both ways." And my inner Mentor, who had never said a single word in any previous process, spoke: "For forty years you have honored every one of these men, and not once did you honor yourself." I became one with my absent brothers, as they lie in their honored glory.

My soul came home.

And I wept.

The Tomb of the Unknown Soldier, located in the National Cemetery at Arlington, Virginia, carries this inscription: "Here lies, in honored glory, an American soldier, known but to God." I honor him and all those I did not know from all wars, who have given their lives in service, affording each his or her honored glory. I honor the Marines of 2nd Platoon, C Company, 1st Battalion, 9th Marine Regiment, 3rd Marine Division, who lost their lives in the Republic of Vietnam. They are known to me and will live in honored glory within my heart for all eternity.

The Journey has *"given"* me nothing. Yet recently during a pilgrimage to India, with fellow Journey Practitioners, while in Rishikesh I immersed myself in the Ganga (Ganges River), a very sacred river. Worshipers bathe daily in its waters for ritual purification, and we were there to do the same. As I stepped in, I was immediately struck by the icy cold of the river, which originates from a glacier high in the Himalayas. I began to sob, as all the guilt about Vietnam came rushing back. My hot tears merged with these frigid waters, and a healing salve was created. All feeling of cold disappeared. I stayed in the water for many minutes, and I sobbed without control. When I had finally emptied my tears, I stepped from the river. I was cleansed, as if all that blood, shed so long ago by my brother Marines, had finally been washed from me. The river had given me what I refused to give myself, forgiveness.

And I wept.

The Journey has *"given"* me nothing. Yet after facilitating a profound process with another beautiful feminine soul, she hugged me, put her head on my chest and said, "I wish you were my dad," filling me with the sacred love between father and daughter, bonding me forever with the daughter of my heart. I knew then that Noreen was not a loss, she was a gift, a truly Divine Gift.

And I wept.

The Journey has *"given"* me nothing. Yet I did a Journey process in which my mom stood in the center of a room. She began to move toward me, one step at a time, and with each step she stopped and said, "I knew you were crying, even though I couldn't be there." I kept pulling my legs back, clenching my jaw and stiffening my body, all classic reactions of an abandoned child. Finally, Mom stood directly over me and said, "I knew when you stopped crying, even though I wasn't there." Then she embraced me, pulling my head into her stomach, into her womb, and I felt her grief for her lost children and her mother's love for me, her child.

I had a flashback to a bleak day, the day I left for the Marine Corps and the eventual war in Vietnam. That morning, April 23, 1964, I kissed my mother on the cheek, told her that I would see her in a few months and left. This day, in this process, I did something I had not done on that day. I embraced her and said, "I love you, Mom."

And I wept.

The Journey has *"given"* me nothing. And yet a prayer to be comfortable, spoken in a prayer circle during a Manifest Abundance retreat, became an outpouring of grief for MaryEllen in a West Virginia cave, less than a month later. When asked afterward how I felt, I replied that I was comfortable, and then remembered what I had prayed for.

And I wept.

The Journey has *"given"* me nothing. Yet during a Journey process with my father, I opened into the pain he felt at trying to be both parents to a little boy, because my mother was very ill. It was the same pain *I* felt at having to be both parents to three young boys when I was widowed. This pain blossomed into an all-consuming sorrow, an emotion that

I don't recall ever having felt before. It continues to flow when tears will come unasked, and it bathes another spot on my soul.

Also during this process, I was asked to open into the Consciousness of Conflict, and discover Conflict's identity. It had become my soul brother from conception. When asked what Conflict wanted, "Just to rest" was the reply, and my father's blessing filled my being.

I was then asked to invite another brother, but there was none there, just a sister whom I had ignored. Asked what her identity was, "Love" was my reply. I then welcomed Love—and what came was my feminine side, and I knew a mother's love for her children.

And I wept.

The Journey has *"given"* me nothing. Yet I had had a strain in my relationship with Nancy. Even changing the wedding vow to MaryEllen had not eased that strain. In a process, a second vow arose, one that I had uttered beneath my breath on that long-ago wedding day, "I will love you, and only you." I never expected her to die first. The process changed the vow, because it no longer served, and a new ease came between Nancy and me. But there was still a specter between us, a palpable presence that I could not release, for I had never let MaryEllen go on with her transition. She was always there, just out of sight, just out of hearing, the barrier that held me away from Nancy. I feared the loss, had never really allowed that West Virginia grief to completely integrate its comfort into my being.

In a further process I was able to free both myself and MaryEllen from those contractive emotions that used to keep us bound together. And I received MaryEllen's blessings to hold my love for Nancy as sacred as any love I have ever felt. When the process ended and I opened my eyes, the facilitator sat there with tears streaming down her face. She said, "MaryEllen stood right here and said to tell you she is now free, too."

And I wept.

I have gotten nothing from The Journey, unless you count finding connection, forgiveness, love, redemption and salvation.

In truth, I have gotten nothing from The Journey; it never was a process of addition but rather one of subtraction—a subtraction of guilt, rage, painful vows that had shackled me in a prison of my own making. Once these oaths were removed, I realized all I sought was already there in the first place, located in my soul. I was shown a path that went from my thinking mind to my essence, a guided tour that found the blighted areas within me and made them oases for myself.

If beauty lies in the eye of the beholder, then that which is sacred resides in the soul.

And about guilt: I don't live there anymore.

I feel great today, alive, vibrant, one with the mountain, rugged, splendid and white-capped with wisdom. I didn't always feel this way. I didn't always *feel*.

I have been to war. I have been numb. I have lived in hatred and rage, fear and pain, conflict and confusion. Now, there is peace.

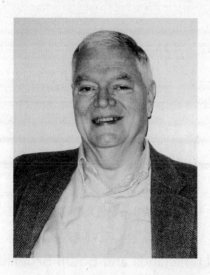

Joe Doyle *and his wife, Nancy, also a Journey Practitioner, live in southern Virginia. Joe is a former business executive who served as an infantryman in the United States Marine Corps and is a veteran of the Vietnam War. He was eyewitness to the events of 9/11 in New York City. This tragedy brought the realization that trauma and conflict are not limited to just military veterans; we all suffer from post-traumatic stress. PTS is a wounding of the soul, not a disorder, and we store each wounding in our repressed cell memories. Joe can be reached by email at marinegrunt2@hotmail.com.*

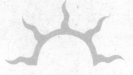

6

Partnership in Truth

by Lumananda and Bodhi Brouillette

LUMI:

I had what I guess you would call a "normal" childhood. What exactly that means, or is, I can't say. My mom and biological father split up when I was young, and when I was four, my mom married a man who adopted me and raised me as his own. He already had three girls by his first wife, and so I became number four. The only difference is that I lived with Mom and him, and the other girls didn't.

I don't remember being unhappy until I was around twelve years old. Things really started shifting then. I was no longer interested in giving my dad manicures or combing his hair all different ways for hours. I was an early bloomer and had left behind the dolls and little-girl things he had so enjoyed. I was growing up, and that led to hormones, opinions, boys and the like, and as I was the youngest, it certainly felt like I was paying for all the things my older sisters had done.

My dad, a wonderful, bighearted man, was also a man who lived in fear, fear that controlled his life. It was a fear that appeared so big, so real for him. I used to say that if worrying were an Olympic sport, my dad would win the gold every time. His fear, with no known way to express itself, came out as anger, yelling and control. It felt oppressive, so oppressive that I used to pray for Mom and Dad to divorce. For years and years I prayed, to no avail. And so the iron fist of control ruled our household, and there were no gray areas; everything was black or white, right or wrong. Control over who ate the last donut, who did what and when, who was to blame, what emotions were acceptable, my curfew, my telephone habits, my social life; even my mom was emotionally "punished" each time she went out of town on business. I began to shrink down more and more, to hide from his notice.

I remember one night I was in trouble for something, I can't even remember what, as I had grown used to not being able to live up to his standards and rules. Anyway, I was in trouble and crying. I remember climbing the stairs to go to my room, and somehow it came out that I was afraid of him. (I pretty much lived in fear of my dad; even though he never touched me, I was very, very afraid of him.) I remember him asking me if I really *was* afraid of him, and I said yes. His response was that I wouldn't have to be afraid of him if I wasn't so bad. I asked him if he still loved me when I was bad, and he said no.

Okay, here it is, something I carried with me for years and years: "If I want to be loved, I have to be good, but I'm not. I'm bad." I was constantly trying to BE GOOD, and always falling short, never good enough to be loved.

Added to this were two very strong ego patterns that had been driving me for years. The first had been put into place just after birth; it's a pattern of perfectionism. Always striving for it, never attaining it. The constant efforts to do things to be perfect affected the way I looked, the way I kept my house, my work, my actions, my possessions, everything, and none of it was ever good enough. Ever. Added to the impossibly high standards I set for myself were the expectations and standards I held others to, and the ever-present judge and jury were there to let me know just how badly I and the others in my world had failed in every moment, every day. The second pattern, set in place for me around age eleven, was of passive-aggressive nonconfrontational behavior, being a peacekeeper if you will. Interesting blend, isn't it? A judgmental perfectionist who at all costs must not rock the boat . . .

I continued through life, making a few friends, falling in love, stepping in and out of marriages and relationships, all the while always working so very hard to be a good girl, do everything right; be who my partner, parents, friends and employers wanted me to be, always living in fear of being found out, because I really wasn't who I was pretending to be.

In my mid- to late twenties, I embarked on a spiritual quest. I knew there was more to life than the existence I'd

been having up to this point. I was even able to *almost* remember a connection, or some kind of knowing, that this
human experience is not all there is, not Who We Really
Are. So I started investigating, dipping a toe in here and
there, searching for something that would speak to me,
something that would touch my heart. I looked at Reiki,
massage, Buddhism, all sorts of things. A lot of them had a
piece or two that resonated, but there were none that made
my heart sing, none that brought me a sense of lightness
and ease.

Then came a September day in 2001. I was in the library,
looking at new releases, and the book *The Journey*, by Brandon Bays, seemed to jump off the shelf at me. I all but heard
it say, "Read me, read me!" I took the book home and starting reading, never realizing the impact it would have on my
life, never realizing that my life would be completely transformed by it! It took me only one day to read the book and
start the adventure of my life.

I read the book the same month it had been released in
America. I asked my partner to read it, or to at least do the
process with me that's in the back of the book, and he really
had no interest. So I put it away. *The Journey* rested in me for
three years, until I encountered a stranger who mentioned
in passing that she'd attended Journey events before and had
done the work! I quickly found a way to speak with her and
asked if there were ever any events in our area, only to find
out there was a Journey Intensive scheduled that month!
Wow! That event, which I promptly registered for, not
only spoke to my heart, it made it sing. Here was what I'd

been looking for! Within three weeks, I was enrolled in the Practitioner Program, which wasn't available in the United States yet, so off I went to the United Kingdom for training. Three trips in three months for the advanced courses, and *lots* of clearing-out happened; life was transforming in so many ways. And there was more to come.

In August of 2005, I was at work at the hair salon, and while having a deep philosophical conversation, I heard myself say, "Okay, I'm ready, I'm ready to be as free as I can be while still walking around in a physical body. I don't care what it takes, I don't care what the cost." The voice in my head asked me if I was sure. I replied, "Yes, I'm sure. I don't care what it takes or what it costs. I'm ready." The voice said, "Well, strap in, then," and so began the ride that continues to this day.

Was it easy? No. Was it comfortable? No. Were there costs? Oh yes. Would I change any of it? Would I take it back if I could? Absolutely not!

In November 2005, the relationship with my life partner ended, to the surprise of both of us. This was the person I had looked forward to being with forever, relishing the idea of spending the rest of my life with him. He was perfect for me, or so I thought. The truth is that a force larger than me had orchestrated the split; I heard words coming out of my mouth, knowing it was the right thing, and being crushed beyond belief. In the three and a half years following, I discovered and let go of so many blocks, beliefs and even vows, things I now believe I wouldn't have been able to release if I had stayed with him.

In April 2006, I had the most amazing Journey process to date. I experienced the death of old patterns, old ways of being, old stories and, more important, "ME." I actually saw the death of who I thought I was, who I held myself to be, letting go of the life I had with my former partner, letting go of the need to control, the passive-aggressiveness, everything! Just letting go of *everything*! Gone were the physical body and the knowledge of how it works. It was like I had just been dropped into this form and had to figure out how to make it work, starting from square one. I can only imagine that an old soul arriving here as a newborn might feel the same way. It was terrifying and exhilarating at the same time; I felt like the phoenix rising from the flames; in fact, I *was* the phoenix! All the old pain, gone . . . and the Truth of Who I Really Am was not only revealed but also directly experienced in a way that can never be hidden again. The fierce love of Truth was remembered.

In 2006, I traveled again to England for an advanced course. During this three-day retreat, even more fell away, leaving me resting as the sublime bliss that is Truth, and from that, a new name was birthed for me, Lumananda, meaning "the bliss of illumination." That light shines brighter and brighter as I continue to look inward, to clear out anything that may be obscuring Truth. Everything is welcome, even the uncomfortable, and it's all good! It's so yummy and delicious to realize Truth—the Truth in me, in you, in all of us—to see through the lies and illusions, to step out of the box that we ourselves and others have fashioned for us. It's extraordinary to soar on the currents of freedom, joy, love and abundance, to awaken to what's real: the infinite potential, infinite possibility, infinite beings we really are.

BODHI:

My father is a large, strong man who through his own experience as a child was taught to rule with an iron fist. He ran his house and family the only way he knew how, with control and violence. Although he may not have known that the emotional and physical pain he was passing on to his four children and wife was even happening, it *did* happen, and it happened big.

The rules that were put into place seemed natural and normal. I didn't even know that it was not normal for a young boy not to be allowed to cry; I thought it was normal to get smacked on the head or slapped in the face for crying, or to be called a baby. It never occurred to me that the threat of having my legs broken, or my head knocked in, didn't happen in every family. I never realized that when my friends were told they could not do something, they were allowed to ask, "Why?" without getting beaten with a belt. In my house, in my family it was just the way it was.

My mother, on the other hand, was a person who did not like conflict and would do whatever she had to in order to avoid it. The famous words of Barbara Brouillette: "Wait until your father gets home." When he did, she left, and the wrath of Glenn Brouillette would wield its ugly hand, belt or coat hanger, and there would be hell to pay.

My mother loved me more than anything. I felt like I was

her favorite of the four of us. I was the youngest, three years from my only sister, five and six years from my older brothers. Mom gave her best to the family, and as a child of an alcoholic father, her mother having worked night shift in a bar for twenty-five years to support the family, she became the caretaker of her four siblings. It was all she would know for the rest of her life: serving others with the fear of not being loved ran through her very existence. Until the day she died in November of 2009, her life never belonged to her.

Seeing life from a perspective of violence and punishment, it would seem very unlikely that we would be members of the church. Yet we went to church every Sunday and did all the things that looked like we were a happy family: church outings, Boy Scouts, Girl Scouts, father-and-son campouts, Little League, soccer, the whole nine yards. What a farce it was. The threats would happen before church, and then the execution would take place when we would get home. I remember when my father threw a fork across the dinner table with such force that it stuck in my brother's chest . . . this within an hour of coming home from taking the Lord's Sacrament and committing our lives to Him one more time.

Fear ran fiercely through the halls of the Brouillette home, and I seemed to get the brunt of the trickle-down effect. As my siblings would acquire my father's rage, they would turn it on me. A vicious cycle, if you will: as they carried out their sentence of pain on me, my father would hear my bellows and attack again, for violence was not allowed in our home! It was the ultimate hypocrisy.

We had a myriad of beliefs about sin in our family, disguised as the strict doctrine of a dogmatic system within our faith. I would comply, or else God would not be pleased. I would have to answer for my sins, and as time went by, the more sins that occurred, the fiercer the punishment. My everlasting soul would not be able to live with the family for time and all eternity. There was another place for me.

I would soon be on a lifelong search for that place. It was Hell, and I was on my way.

It was baptism time; the young children of our church are baptized when they turn eight years old. The age of accountability, they say, and I was turning eight. I didn't realize my life would be forever changed with a few decisions and the actions that would follow. The only thing I knew about being baptized was that when my father dunked me into the water, my sins would be washed away; everything I did wrong prior to that moment would no longer be on the Naughty List that God was keeping up in Heaven. It would be erased, and then another list would start, a list that would never be erased. It would be with me until I died; after that, God would decide if I lived with Him or would I live in everlasting punishment.

The sins I feared the most were: (1) not obeying the Word of Wisdom, and (2) lying to my parents. Although it was a standard practice of mine to lie, the fear of being caught was fierce, so I had to be good at it. The Word of Wisdom was a set of principles that dated from the 1800s: no smoking, no drinking alcohol, tea or coffee, no excessive eating of meats, etc. In my home it went even further, as we could not have any caffeine, no Coca-Cola or Pepsi.

It was the Friday before my baptism; I can still remember the excitement when I received a birthday card in the mail, and in it was a check for ten dollars from my grandmother Emily. Wow! Ten dollars was a lot of money, and I could buy a lot of things. What I wanted most was an RC Cola. There was a contest: if you popped the cap and peeled the plastic cover off from underneath the cap, you could win a prize.

The baptism came and went, and it was now Monday afternoon; I found myself with check in hand heading down to the store to buy the RC Cola. Not remembering the contract that I had made with Jesus just two days before, I walked into the store, picked up the bottle—and suddenly realized that what I was about to do was a sin. But for some reason, my obsession with the bottle-cap game was so strong that it didn't matter. I purchased the cola and put it in a brown paper sack; with the sack in hand I went out to the back of the store and hid behind a Dumpster. Taking the cola out of the bag, I remember saying, "I should not do this," yet again the obsession was so strong that I popped the cap using the edge of the Dumpster. As I picked up the cap from the ground, I pulled the plastic cover. I can still see the words "Sorry Try Again."

Disappointment consumed me. I looked at the full bottle of cola and said to myself, "It's here; I might as well drink it."

In that instant, with that decision, my life changed forever. I took the bottle and placed it to my lips, and as I took the first drink I thought to myself, "I am going to Hell," clear as a summer day. I thought, "Don't waste it, you're going to Hell anyway," so I continued to drink. This was the start of a pattern that would stay with me for the next thirty-seven years.

The pattern started playing out almost immediately. I hid the sin from my parents, Sunday school teachers, bishop and everyone else in my life. It felt as though there was a dark cloud in and around me, and I had to hide it. All the lies and strategies that were born from that secret created even more painful patterns that would shatter the life of a little boy. I couldn't take it any longer; the pain was too great; there had to be a way for me not to feel! Finding ways of not feeling wasn't a mystery to me, but this pain was beyond anything I had ever experienced up to this point in my life.

At the age of nine years I found myself in a small central California town, another bottle in hand. This time it was not RC Cola; it was Southern Comfort whisky. How ironic that the name of the first drink of alcohol I would take included the word *comfort*. It spoke to me like a long-lost friend, a friend that would stay with me, protect me and love me for the next fourteen years. I placed the bottle of whisky to my lips and euphoria arrived. No more sin, no more secret; it all fell away. All the pains of my father's beatings and insults would no longer control me. I was free at last.

The problem was that the whisky ran out; I was only nine, and it was not easy to get. There had to be another way! I soon realized there was. Watching my brother's friend as he held a plastic bag up to his mouth, I saw him begin to sway back and forth and then fall to the ground. I picked up the bag and smelled the aroma of some sort of glue; it was clear and it smelled of chemicals. I took a deep breath in and numbness settled throughout my body. Again euphoria had arrived. This time I found that I could stop the pain any time I wanted to; glue, paint, and gas from a gas can were all it took.

Then came LSD at age eleven, marijuana, cocaine, PCP and the final frontier of meth. Six years of using meth on a daily basis. Sleeping only eight hours in one month, weighing 130 pounds with a 26-inch waist, my life was on an autopilot search to be rid of all feeling. I spent close to five of those fourteen years behind bars, learning how to live my life with my truest essence hiding behind hate, shame, guilt and rage. I created a life where I could manipulate people to take care of me and give me food, shelter, clothes and the like. And I was sure my wish would soon be accomplished: I would die and be with the evils to be.

Then on February 17, 1989, I ran out of people to take care of me and found myself in a meeting of Alcoholics Anonymous. I had never heard of it before, and yet there I was. Earlier that day would be the last time I would take any kind of mood-altering substances for the next nineteen years. I sobered up and thought my life would get better; however, it only got worse. The feelings came, they came in droves, and without the use of drugs or alcohol there was nowhere to turn. A seventeen-year depression fell upon me. I could barely function in this world of lack and hate. Again another way had to be found not to feel.

I turned to AA, spending every hour I could in meetings and coffee shops. Finding people who were just like me, who did not want to feel, I created a community of friends who would cosign my crap as I marched through this life again with all the pain and suffering of a man without hope. As AA stopped working for me, a myriad of strategies took its place: gambling, softball, religion, sex and many, many more. And the feelings kept coming. The more they came, the more I ran.

In November 2005, I ran myself into a book called *The Journey,* written by Brandon Bays. Reading was not something *I* did, it was something *others* did, and I was not privy to that kind of commitment or perseverance. Up to that point in my life I had read only five books, but I felt very different about this book and Brandon's story. I read it in one night; it was amazing to hear how someone could heal in such a way. However, I didn't know how this book could help *me.* I put the book back on the shelf and did not give it a thought for another ten months.

Then I ran into the same friend who gave me the book, and she told me about a workshop that was going to be here the next weekend. I had no money; in fact I was $50,000 in debt. I felt hopeless; she told me how her story of hopelessness turned into gratitude and love. I found the money, and on Saturday, September 16, 2006, my life changed forever.

I spent the next three days feeling more emotions than I had in my entire life. And inside those emotions was a sense of freedom that I never knew existed. The amount of love that I felt from Skip Lackey, the presenter of the workshop, had never been a part of my knowing. He shared with me that I never had to run. That all the answers were within me, hiding behind all the lies, strategies and games that got put into place from years of fear. And I finally discovered that these three days of really feeling my emotions had actually been *less* painful than all the strategies I had used in a lifetime of running from my pain.

Freedom called me to my Self; it showed me a glimpse of who I truly am. I had to have more. But how? I put an intention out to the universe and vowed that whatever I needed to do to awaken to this amazing truth that I felt, I would do. I had no idea what that would be; the prayer was so fierce that it didn't matter.

I scrimped and saved every penny I had; I would even borrow money to get myself to the next Journey event. I applied for the Practitioner Program and was accepted. I didn't apply so that I could help others; I just knew that I had to open and realize all the ways that my life had been held back by my own beliefs. And when the money was gone and it looked as if there was no way for me to complete the program, I received a phone call from the Journey office: a beautiful couple had gifted me with the rest of the program.

Because of this amazing work and the courageous people who have forged the path before me and so freely given to me what grace has given to them, my life has been forever changed. There is no more looking outside of me for answers that have always been there inside. The truth has always been here, it's here now and it can't leave. I have embodied gratitude with the essence of my entire being; there is a knowing that the story of my past is only that: A STORY, not real. There is a blessed awareness of this moment, and then this moment and then this one. Feeling the grace of the oneness of all, in each moment, creates the most amazing recognition of truth that I have ever experienced. For all of you who are seeking the freedom that seems to escape you . . . I can only say, "STOP, and know that you are already FREE, you are already WHOLE, you are already TRUTH." Be still and know that You Are!

LUMI:

Life was wonderful—full of joy, love, peace, friends, family and new experiences. The only thing that seemed to be "missing" was a life partner. A partner who, as I was fond of saying, would be on his path and be able to support me on mine, someone who didn't have to stand in my fire but would be standing in one of his own. As I put out to grace for this, I was confident I was ready . . . and then some issue would show up, and clear, and I'd realize I hadn't been ready. I'd state it again. Again, an issue would show up, and clear; again the realization. I made a list of what my life partner was like, what our life would be like, how we would be with each other. Then, aaahhhhh, he came, most unexpectedly. Here was someone I'd met through The Journey three or so years before and never imagined would be the partner I'd asked for! I was even his mentor as he went through the Practitioner Program. Wow!

The relationship unfolded so beautifully, gracefully, effortlessly and quickly! Our first date was a Wednesday in late April, and we were married just eighteen weeks later. We both just knew this was what we'd been asking for: the opportunity to live and love in Truth, in relationship. Do we "trigger" each other? Yes. Sometimes something one of us says or does (or doesn't!) triggers emotion, old patterns and behaviors. Do anger, fear and hurt show up? Absolutely, and we're honest about that. We know, each of us, that when things happen, if it sticks, if one of us feels the zing, it's ours. Not the other's fault or responsibility. Do we honor our commitment to Truth? Yes! We stay true to Truth, sharing what's true in that moment. That was and is the basis of our wedding vows, committing ourselves to live in and as Truth, and letting Truth live through us.

This is the most amazing relationship of my life. I've asked for open, honest, heart-centered communication, and it's here! It's beautiful and freeing—amazingly, wonderfully, deliciously freeing!

It's also our joy to share with others the way to Freedom that we've found, so two years ago we started our company, Live-n-Truth. We work with people one-on-one or in groups so they can live the Truth, Freedom, Joy, Infinite Potential and Abundance they really are.

BODHI:

There is a way that Lumi has made me aware of my own series of stories, lies, beliefs, vows and promises. She has allowed me to see the rules that got put into place from the very beginning of my life: rules about how a relationship

should be, how I should treat my partner and how my partner should treat me. She has given me invitations to look
deep into the truth, the terror that has been the underlying
cause of all the relationships within my life that ended with
pain and suffering. She has created a safe place for me to go,
and she is doing this with one principle: "*It's not about me.*"
She knows it's not about her: that all my pain comes from
my own story of past experiences. And she lets me have
them, and allows everything to be present, even if there
seems to be blame or victimization here.

Never once in my past was I able to be truly honest with
my partner, only because honesty has come to me in stages.
I believed myself to be honest at the time; I was as honest
as I could be. The real truth is that I could not differentiate
the true from the false that had ruled my life. Beliefs and
promises that I have made created patterns that told me that
it was not safe to love, and that in no way was I worthy of
being loved. These old patterns would not let me see the
truth of who I am. Blaming others for my own insecurities,
lashing out as I became the victim of my own worst stories,
I would try desperately to control the very thing that wants
to be set free.

My intimate life has been consumed by a double-binding
belief that said, on the one hand, "I would rather die than
be alone," and on the other hand, "I am truly not worthy of
being loved; I am a monster, a man who does not know how
to love, a man incapable of loving." I have seen over and over
again on this path of self-awareness that the fear of dying
alone paralyzed me and depleted my very desire to have a

companion. The very thing that I was afraid of most was always with me: that the cage would break and the monster would escape, destroying all in its path—and it had the power to destroy lives, others' and mine.

As this work has shown up in my life, it has taken all of me, in all ways, and it is especially true in my intimate relationships. My love for this Truth has been realized even more fully in the beautiful relationship that has blossomed with my beloved Lumi. Our wedding vows were simply put: "We honor truth, we will commit ourselves to truth, whatever truth might be. We will tell the truth, we will spend our time together being in authentic conversation. We promise to honor what the universe is sharing with us, and what it will share with us in the future. We will follow the bread crumbs."

It seems highly unlikely that two people who have come from two such opposite worlds should find each other. It is beyond anything that my mind can envision; there is a love that has been realized within us that sees the other as pure and whole. We have fallen deeply in love and have created a world of authentic love and true companionship. We have recognized that the very differences we have experienced in our lives are what have created this stunning connection of oneness. Our passion is to share this with anyone who would like to live in a true and conscious relationship.

LUMI AND BODHI:

And so life just continues to flower, to blossom open and sow its seeds of freedom. It doesn't seem real, that old story of pain and suffering, and it isn't. What *is* real just *is* . . . it is who we are under the layers of old beliefs, expectations and pain. We are all that is and all that isn't. We just Are.

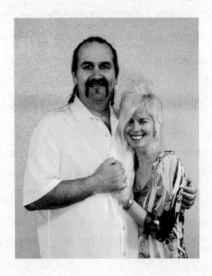

Lumananda and Bodhi Brouillette *are internationally Accredited Journey Practitioners. Bodhi is also a certified Visionary Leadership Coach. They are owners of Live-n-Truth out of Boulder, Colorado, specializing in the process of helping others find and release limiting beliefs that have caused physical, emotional and mental suffering. For more information, please go to www.liventruth.com.*

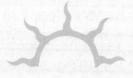

7

The Coping Game

by Bet Diening-Weatherston

"I'm sure glad we cut that mole off, Bet," said my doctor, "because you've got melanoma!"

What???!

How does a person who is surrounded by a loving family, who lives in the most beautiful place on the planet, who eats organically and who is physically active get such a life-threatening form of cancer? I'm the one sitting in the shade with a hat on, for God's sake . . . it makes no sense at all!

Until I looked at the way I stuffed my emotions . . .

The fierceness of emotions has always taken my breath away. Emotions overwhelm me—it's as if the circuitry in my body and mind blitz out, clamping my throat shut, stealing my words. Having "control" over my feelings meant I just might not fall apart in public . . . or in private, for that matter. *And* my gut knew that I couldn't go on living this way.

One of my mom's mantras was, "Make somebody else happy so that you can be happy!" I remember feeling that it was my job to keep everybody happy, all six billion of them, so that I could rest, feel peace and reassure myself that life wasn't too scary to experience wholeheartedly. It felt like an impossible job—and yet I took on this task with such passion and conviction that it took melanoma smacking me over the head to make me pay attention . . . to me!

My dad, on the other hand, reminded me that for me to take care of my needs was "selfish—and there are enough selfish people on the planet, thank you very much!" So, as you may appreciate, the double whammy set me up for running around hoping to save all of humanity—except, of course, myself.

My parents are beautiful people, well intentioned, conditioned by their birth families, society and life, and they truly felt that they were guiding us to our highest and best. Unfortunately, I never questioned the truth of their words, nor their impact on me and others, until I stopped long enough to notice what I was really experiencing at the core of my being.

I was born December 15, 1960, the last of eight kids, to a family who had recently emigrated from Holland. My mom was five months pregnant with me when the entire entourage packed up their belongings and moved into a two-bedroom bungalow in Don Mills, Ontario. My parents felt that Canada would be the proverbial land of opportunity for all of us children. I'm pretty sure that my experience of this move-while-in-utero was a chemical soup of fear, anxiety, sadness, excitement and overwhelm. It seems to me that I was born scared, with a visceral need to take care of everyone else so that *I* would start to feel safe and connected.

I remember at a very young age being absolutely petrified of not being able to figure out "time," where the universe began and ended, what the purpose of being born was. Who was God, and fundamentally who was "I"? Whenever I read a book that had the word *God* in it I would put my finger over it (I'd already read it, though!) so as not to start this obsessive thinking again and again. The mind is a master game player, and mine was on overdrive.

There are some Dutch expressions that are relevant to the strategies I adopted in order to cope with this terror, since being this afraid was not tolerated. (The Dutch are good at this coping game.) The gist of the messages I learned from my culture was basically to get over myself and to accept that *there were no definitive answers*, no matter how hard I tried to figure this all out. Not that this advice helped at all. I would still lie in bed, eyes wide open, in a cold sweat, trying not to feel the phenomenal vastness of the universe, which scared the soul out of me. I even made a deal with my sister that as long as she would groan out a response now and again, I would keep talking until I fell asleep. It never worked; she was out cold by the time her head hit the pillow, and I was forced to face the terrifying abyss alone.

I remember asking my dad, asking a priest, asking a minister, asking just about anybody I could engage with, to give me the answers . . . I needed the answers . . . I was desperate for the answers . . . so I could get some sleep. Nobody had them. How could this be? The question haunted me.

Stubborn, and determined to get some relief from the terror, I chose another way to cope: as well as a seeker, I became an athlete. I figured out that when I got myself so unbelievably tired that my body would crash out in exhaustion, my mind would be robbed of any opportunity to engage in this game called "Who Am I?" By now I was about seven years old and had already created a plethora of strategies to avoid the intensity of emotions. And soon after that I applied the best strategy of all: I became an observer of life and a voice for others, not myself—the one who "has it all together" and can look on from the sidelines with a faint smile of superiority on her face . . .

I learned that it wasn't safe to feel, that feelings set me up for ridicule, and that meant there was no way in hell my emotions were going to come to the surface for all to see. Except, of course, when I got embarrassed and my face would turn beet red. I learned that my body had a mind of its own and would expose me to others, and expose my game to myself, without my permission . . . it felt like a traitor. I was so keen to control the inner workings of the body, so that the world would buy my façade of "having it together." What a joke!

I also learned to use humor to cope. Some of the best guffaws I've had were during the most intense moments, when the emotions I felt were over the top. Laughing life away seemed to shave off the pointy edges, making existence more palatable and ultimately safe. Humor, tinged with sarcasm or mixed with a flavor of self-deprecation, helped keep me believing that I was at the helm of my experiences and not at the whim of life's cruel jokes.

I learned that I cared too much, loved too much, worried too much about things I had no control over. It was an exhausting way to experience life, as I was constantly stuffing down how I truly felt in the hopes that I wouldn't have to experience it fully.

One of my other jobs in life was to "fix" everybody, as it was clear in our birth family that *we* had our act together and the rest of the world was broken. Now, please remember that our family was working with the best tools we had at the time, and it never occurred to me that this concept was completely flawed. So I set about fixing the world, having noticed (from the sidelines) that there were patterns that constantly repeated themselves.

Imagine how happy people were to learn from me that they could use some tweaking . . . if only they could see how much better they'd feel once they'd changed! I remember a boss of mine, exasperated, stating once, "Sure, you can quit working for me and go someplace else—only to meet another 'me' at your next job and set up the same problems." It was the classic example of, "No matter where you go, there you are!" Finally, I began to realize that the common thread to my problems and conflicts was *me*.

Good intentions be damned . . . I was at the core of my own upheaval. I began to realize that perhaps the "Diening" way wasn't the only way, and probably not the best way, to be. Cam, my husband, is a patient man, and over the past twenty-eight years has been trying to point out that maybe, just maybe, there are other opinions out there that work just fine. That it's none of my business how the rest of the human race is doing, nor is it my right to advise humanity on how to get its act together.

I sometimes cringe at my own arrogance. I am thoroughly embarrassed, and it makes me blush to wonder how many people I have railroaded or derailed in life. Thank Life for Forgiveness!

Soon after acknowledging that it was me causing my own grief, and after learning that I had in-situ melanoma, I was introduced to Brandon Bays's book, *The Journey*. It intrigued me and pulled me in . . . and being an experiential learner, I decided to travel to Ottawa to join a small group of my family members at this enormously, overwhelmingly, phenomenally emotional Journey Intensive. Holy #@$!

My first process had me matched me up with a gentleman who had experienced my worst nightmare . . . the death of his child sixteen years before. I choked my way through "his" process, clinging to the script like a lifeline to hope . . . hope that he would not be destroyed by the experience and hope that *I* wouldn't implode. It baffles me to this day how we sobbed our way through his pain, his loss, his guilt, his unbelievable grief, to peace and acceptance . . . gifts unfathomable to me. I was gobsmacked by the transition that I witnessed and co-facilitated: from utter despair to elation . . . in a matter of maybe two hours.

My second process taught me another invaluable lesson. The partner who I had for round two was completely disengaged from the experience, and I thought, "Oh man, this is going to be awkward"——me, with an aversion to being emotionally exposed, sharing an intimate experience with what felt like a fence post. And I learned that it really has nothing to do with the other person. That it really is all about me . . . nobody else . . . and that not only is that okay, it is *necessary* to acknowledge that *I am responsible for only my own well-being*. What a relief. I just shaved off 5,999,999,999 other people from my "to do" list.

My third process that weekend offered me yet another "Aha" moment: discovering that at the same time I had been emptying out my unfinished business with my mom in *my* process, *she* was having an almost identical conversation with my sisters around the breakfast table in British Columbia. How could that be?? I used to joke that if there were ever any thought police, I'd get arrested . . . What a lesson to realize that not only do our thoughts travel energetically (5,000 kms), but even the content of the story can be available to the one we are connecting with internally. Yikes!

And so I was hooked, in a good way, on joining the Journey Practitioner Program.

During the Practitioner Program, one of the most profound processes I experienced exorcised an inner vision that had haunted me for almost a decade. About eight years previously, a friend of mine had asked me if I had ever meditated before, and I had said that my attention span didn't allow me to sit long enough to relax. Deep down I knew that meditating would encourage me to feel and see things that I had put under wraps. On that occasion eight years before, though, for whatever reason, I agreed to give it a try.

It makes me weep to this day remembering the vision that had appeared when I got still: *A little two-year-old boy, dressed in a white shirt and dungarees, is swinging his arms like he is an airplane, and I know that he dies in the next scene. In my absolute heart of hearts, I know that if I swivel my head to the right, I will see some catastrophic vision of innocence being wiped off the planet. And I can't force myself to face it.*

I finished my meditation sobbing, not being able to articulate what had just happened. When my friend, connecting with my devastation, said, "I know, I know!" I choked out, "Know *what*?! What was that, and who was that little boy?" And I broke down. Though no such event has occurred in my present lifetime, my gut knew that he was my son in a prior life, and that it was my fault that he died that day.

Not until my Journey process some eight years later did I visit this scene again: *I plunge into grief and sadness as I am invited to turn my head to face what's there. My son, floating with his blond hair, facedown, in a pond, dead! It was on my watch that he died. I didn't protect him from himself, and he drowned. To this day it makes me shudder, the wail that escaped from my soul as I went into the pond and picked up his soaking wet body and begged him for forgiveness. I moaned out that I was so sorry that he died alone, in cold water, while I sat on the grassy hill watching him play. I hurled curses at myself for robbing him of his life due to my negligence. It was my fault that he was gone . . . my son . . . my beautifully gorgeous son.*

Is this memory real? Who knows? Who cares! It feels real! It was definitely a part of my "story," and it explains so much about how I have raised our two sons. I have smothered our boys and kept them close by "just in case." I have said a resounding "NO!" to so many opportunities so that they are nearby and safe. I have controlled their lives so that I can feel like everything's going to be okay, because I wouldn't want to be me if they died. I couldn't go through that experience again.

By the end of this process, I had showered myself with forgiveness and could breathe a little more easily, having let go of the stranglehold that pain had had on my heart. After I left that course, I mourned the loss of this beautiful little being and honored the short time that we shared together. His name was James.

And so I put out a fierce intention to turn and face whatever else lay lurking under the radar, now knowing that there must be more that I had stuffed away. Wow . . . what an invitation to the Universe. That invitation has been fully answered: I have continued to find and let go of the hidden pain running my oh-so-safe, oh-so-vigilant, observing-from-the-sidelines coping game. And now I no longer need to be a spectator in my own life.

Now I am free to be who my soul has wanted me to be. The clarity of my life's purpose, discovered and unraveled during Life Transformation Week (the final course in the Practitioner Program) has helped me figure out at last what I want to be when I grow up! I want to be a being who explores and shares Truth with humility, forgiveness, laughter, love and hope. I have a desire to share these qualities with whoever feels called to clear their "stuff" so that they can live life fully. I want to hang out with those folks who feel the same way I do.

I am now so willing to help co-create a major shift in consciousness for all of us—so willing that it makes my head spin. I have a passion to share these Journey tools, especially with the First Nations Peoples all over the world, most specifically in Canada. I hope to empower others to be their own voice, to laugh more, to play full on and have fun. That's what I want to be/do as I grow up. Finally, I'm not afraid to live anymore.

And so I began to show up . . .

As part of the Practitioner Program, we are required to do forty-five case studies. I remember two very profound experiences that have been etched into my being.

First, I worked with a woman who was terminally ill with cancer. For me to actually step into the room of a dying patient is a testament to this work in itself. I would *never* have dreamed that possible for me, to welcome this kind of shift to occur . . .

I started by sharing with my client that death scared the heck out of me and that I was willing to work through my own fears with her. I asked her if she *would be willing* to allow me the honor of being with her as she turned and faced her fears.

We shared four lovely sessions together before she died, and this is what I learned: she was brave; she was curious to discover what gifts lay in the tumors; she did not give up hope; she was incredibly grateful for our times together as she came to terms with family and friends, opening doors that had been previously shut. She died peacefully in the company of her family, from whom she had been estranged. At her deathbed I noticed that she wore a thumb ring, and it struck me that there was a way to honor her and to remind myself to be grateful for all that life has on offer. So I too now wear such a ring.

This is what I learned about myself: I showed up, four times, and once more in her palliative care room, two days before she passed on. I was at peace with myself, with life and especially with the little boy who drowned. I realized that I had an inner strength that I hadn't credited myself with and I knew that I'd be okay . . . that our sons would be okay . . . that six billion people on the planet would thrive, even without my help.

The other incredibly profound experience I had while leading a Journey process was when I seemed to step viscerally into a client's memory. The scenes were vivid, the emotions unbelievably intense, and the terror breathtaking. All I could do was be a witness to this event. It was like being part of a movie and not being able to do a thing to stop it, change it or to be protected from the battle that ensued. My whole body engaged in somebody else's life story, albeit from the sidelines, and bore witness to the atrocities of their memories.

My client moved through that memory only to experience many more during our session together. It felt like we were on a scavenger hunt, collecting up meaningful lessons that could be applied, with clarity and assuredness, to this life stream. To this day, she remains focused and joyful about her contributions to society.

And still I knew there was more . . .

When Kevin Billett, Brandon Bays's husband and CEO of The Journey worldwide, announced that he was going to start a Visionary Leadership series, I misunderstood and thought that he was going to target companies and corporations, which held no interest for me whatsoever. The part that I misunderstood was that it held no interest for me.

I remember peeking through the crack of the door during their first introductory meeting and wondering when the meeting was going to be over so that I could "play" with those in attendance. My gut kept saying, "Bet, you know you should be in there," and I tootled off smugly telling my gut to take a rest. Enough with clearing blocks and limiting beliefs already . . . What about integrating the past year and a half's experiences and just coasting for a while?

Nope, not meant to be!

I can't clearly remember how I ended up sitting in the audience at the first Visionary Leadership course; somehow my body and being knew to show up. Of course, once you start something, you may as well go whole hog, and so I bounded into the entire four-part program.

Here's where I learned: that there is no room for hiding out from yourself or your audiences, as you stand in complete exposure on stage, speaking from passion and Truth. At one point I remember using humor to deflect how I was really feeling during my soliloquy in front of twenty-plus people, and Kevin had me stop and start again. Geesh! It's amazing how the body knows to stay put, to try again, to honor itself in the name of leadership instead of bolting for the door in shame.

Partway through the Leadership series, Kevin offered five one-day sessions for anyone interested in sharing a day with him as coach. It was like somebody had catapulted me up onto the stage, and before I could stop the words from spilling out of my mouth, I asked him if he'd be willing to share one of those days with me . . . the eighth of eight kids . . . the little one—and he said, "Sure, I'd love to!" And, ever the eloquent speaker, I said, "Really!?"

Now, I'm not one to go ga-ga over other people, and I had a hard time figuring out why he'd said yes. So I dove into my Journey tool kit and did some process work on not feeling good enough, not screwing up, not wasting anybody's time, making the most of the opportunity and whatever else I could think of that would honor his generous gift.

It changed my life . . .

We met and had coffee at Starbucks, where Kevin gently elicited what was going on in my world at the time. My friend's husband had just passed away. I was incapacitated by her grief, as I was witness to the love they so openly shared and felt their overwhelming sadness as his body gave way to cancer. And I knew that the love and sadness I was feeling were not theirs but my own. I also knew that I wanted to face this grief so that I could be of service to others who faced the same intensity of emotions.

During my day with Kevin, he asked me if I was good at asking for help, and I snapped my head up and said, "Nope!"

"Okay," he responded, "*Would you be willing* to make a 'Can't List' of the things you can't ask help for, and who you can't ask this help from, and then go and ask them?"

I thought, "Are you serious?"

During our conversation over coffee, I shared some of my teaching history and how being in the Arctic had been an "everything" experience. Some of the life lessons I had learned while working with the Inuit were profoundly simple to me. Kevin, moved, said I had inspired him to suggest that I become involved with the Social Certification Program in Canada. My tongue and mind got all twisted up; very ineloquently I announced that I didn't want *him* to be inspired and me dependent on *his* inspiration, as he was then in control of whether or not this opportunity would come to fruition. I wanted to be inspired by inspiration itself and not by a human being!

Oh boy . . . did I stay awake that night. I was completely embarrassed by how ungracious I'd been to him. He had just given me a day of his time to coach me, and here I was negotiating about how I wanted the gift to appear. And I couldn't talk to him about it—I just couldn't. I was too ashamed to talk to him and hear his answer. Then I realized that he was the first person on my Can't List. So I decided to show up.

Meeting up with everyone for breakfast the next morning, I asked him if I could walk him to the elevator. I wanted to know if he felt that I had offended him in any way and he immediately said, "No! Of course you want to be inspired by inspiration!" End of story . . . No story . . . No waste of energy wondering if . . . What a relief!

I have used this Can't List tool on many occasions, and it has opened up countless doors and opportunities for me. It is only our perception that we couldn't, shouldn't, wouldn't possibly be able to . . . whatever! I urge you to try it. In some weird, twisted way, it's kind of fun!

Since May 2009, I have been blessed with many opportunities to be "lead trainer" (coordinating the logistics and holding the energetic space for the presenter) at various Journey and Leadership events in both Canada and the United States. At the first such event, I gulped and said, "So does this job come with a manual . . . a how-to?" and was gently told, "Nope, just open to what is needed in the moment." And so I did. And I have loved every experience so far as this work continues to evolve, allowing me to connect more of the dots together in deeper realizations of Truth.

One of the newly created Leadership processes is designed to slice through, with laser-sharp accuracy, a set of stacked limiting beliefs, which rest on a core belief. At the heart of this belief is likely some phobia or plain fear around . . . (you fill in the blank). Mine was death. For my entire life I have been phobic about death . . . mainly others' deaths, as I was afraid that I would plunge into such profound grief that I would stay stuck in this living nightmare. As a result, I have spent forty-nine and a half years strategizing to keep myself, my loved ones and the rest of the folks on the planet safe and alive.

During this process, my partner invited me to feel the enormous terror of death, and immediately I became that seven-year-old little girl again, lying in my bed in a cold sweat. At some point it felt like I was floating out in the vast universe, when my partner asked, "and Who Are You in the vastness?" Off to my left, I noticed a fireball of light that had little sparks of light coming from it. Suddenly I knew that this exquisite globe was Love itself and that the tiny sparks were beings headed off to earth as messengers of this Love . . . and that I was one of them.

I had feared death all of my life, yet what I came to realize is that it's not death that I am afraid of, it's the *fierceness of love* that has had a stranglehold on my heart. When someone or something dies, it is the absence of their *love* that I fear . . . not the death itself. When I turned to face this Love, it obliterated me, shattering me into a million atoms. And I felt peace like never before. I *am* Love. You *are* Love . . . That's really all that matters. Everything else is simply a game of pain, separating us from that which we are at our core . . . *Love.* No wonder I love my family so much . . . and animals, and the planet. It's a love fest!!!

So, back to where we started, with the melanoma. Even though it's true I burn easily because of my skin type, I believe that at the core of this cancer, for me, was a disconnect from this all-encompassing Love . . . the fear of losing this Love through death . . . or of being consumed completely by its ferocity.

I have no intentions of broiling my body with baby oil out in the sun to test this theory, and where the melanoma was found has never seen the light of day . . . so, you decide. In any case, I got the growth surgically removed and felt extraordinarily blessed and mightily relieved that the cancer was contained and the operation a full success.

A very wise practitioner said to me one day, "Bet, you know why you got melanoma?"

Sheepishly, I said, "No."

She said, "You got melanoma because you need to make friends with the sun, you need to tell the sun you love her . . . and spend ten minutes a day facing the sun and absorbing her energy."

How true these words are . . . I choose to turn and face *me*, tell me I love me and spend at least ten minutes a day celebrating my life, in love and in service.

And, so I do . . . I show up in life, I use any and all the tools I can get my awareness connected to, for myself and others. I run through the trails, I crank up the tunes and dance like nobody's watching. I say outrageous things to make myself and others laugh . . . laughing is so good for the soul, I believe it heals all. I make dates with my husband, my sons Jorin and Connor, and I celebrate . . . I live in gratitude even when I'm in a pissy mood, because that too is welcome.

A little while ago I had the privilege of spending a week with Jorin (then eighteen and a half years old) at a cattle ranch in the interior of British Columbia. He'd been studying in Ontario for the past year, and I realized that since he was born we hadn't spent any just-Mom-and-Jorin alone time. So I made this date with him, and it was beautiful.

We were making dinner together when he decided to let me know that he felt that I was abandoning Cam and Connor with all of the traveling that I'd been doing. He expressed quite vehemently that I wasn't there enough for Connor like I should be, and that I needed to go back to how I used to be. Tenderly, I asked him why. He burst into tears, saying, "I miss my mom!" and it broke my heart one more time, as I was sitting right there next to him. I hugged him and said, "I'm right here, Jor. I haven't gone anywhere . . . it's still me. I've just changed in that I am no longer that controlling, crazy lady that you used to know, and it's giving both you and me a lot more freedom." So he expressed how he missed the influence I'd had in shaping his life and was concerned that that guidance wasn't going to be available to Connor. I told him how I missed being the mom to a younger him and how much I had loved that role in his life. By the end of our conversation, he realized that my cutting the stranglehold of control over both my sons actually gave us all more authentic freedom than the games I used to play. He thanked me and honored how happy I am now. I expressed how much more breathing space was available to everyone now that I had worked through major clumps of my fear.

The next morning the Universe would provide us with a concretizing lesson on how this shift played out.

I was reluctant to leave him all alone up on the ranch, in the middle of nowhere, with nobody looking out for him, in the heart of cougar and bear country. Not only was the location dicey, but his job required him to go into the fields to run the irrigation pipes and motors as well as traveling by ATV through vast tracts of land. Oh boy . . . nothing like pushing Mommy's buttons . . . so I tentatively asked him if he'd like me to stay a few days longer so we could continue enjoying each other's company and so that I wouldn't have to worry about him.

Jorin proudly announced that he was going to go it alone and that it was okay for me to go back home to be with Cam and Con. Now, normally I would pretend that everything is fine, that I'm good, and that life is ticking along beautifully . . . no matter how I really felt. This time, the floodgates opened up as I choked out that I would miss him horribly and that I wished him a safe time.

I could hardly see through the tears as I drove down the switchback mountains headed for home. I cried for a good half hour, sobbing my way down the mountain as I felt the umbilical cord stretch to near breaking point, when I noticed a message on my cell. "Mom, if it makes you happy, turn the car around and come on back!" Man, was I tempted, but my gut knew that the best thing for the two of us was for me to hit the gas pedal and to keep heading for the coast. When I spoke with Jorin, I explained that this was exactly what I was talking about. The old me would have raced back and held him tight out of fear and love. Now I was able to continue toward home out of freedom and love. He got it. I got it! And we both survived to learn that in honoring each other's wishes, the world has so many rich experiences for us to learn from.

I asked Connor how he and I could spend some one-on-one time, and he invited me to read a book to him every night . . . just like we did when he was younger. It's amazing how much room a seventeen-year-old kid takes up when lying together compared to when he was tiny . . . and it warms my heart to know that this connection of love still exists, actually never goes away and is constantly available to be shared . . . when we remember.

Cam continues to be unbelievably supportive of my adventures. We've had many a conscious conversation about how he feels in my absence, and, like the boys, he has noticed a fundamental shift in how much happier I am. He misses me, I miss him, and that's perfectly okay. I recognize that it is not my responsibility to make him happy either, and it's my pleasure to grow old together with him as long as life offers us the opportunity. These powerful tools that allow a mom like me to love my family without fear of losing them are a gift beyond measure and one that is a pleasure for me to share with anyone willing to show up in their own lives.

And, so life goes on. Every day is a surprise, a gift, an opportunity to choose to live life in gratitude. Some days are more fun than others, and each day is perfect. The tools that I have learned by becoming an Accredited Journey Practitioner and a Conscious Leadership Coach serve me well. It is my wish to share them with others.

It's a beautiful thing, this Freedom is . . . and it's an invitation for us all to actively choose what we want to experience and offer in life. So, what do *you* want, really, really want, to experience in life? These tools will help you clear away misconceptions and limiting beliefs, allowing you to realize that the best gift in life . . . is you! You are what you seek. Call the search off. You are IT!

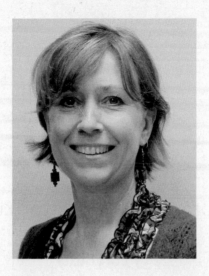

Bet Diening-Weatherston, *her husband, Cam, and two sons, Jorin and Connor, live in a self-built timber-frame home in the rain forests of British Columbia's Sunshine Coast. Bet is a presenter for both The Journey and Visionary Leadership. She is also the Journey Workshop Coordinator for North America. Visit her website at www .wouldyoubewilling.com.*

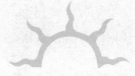

8

From Train Wreck to Truth

by Lori Beaty

When I was a small child, I considered my life and my family to be rather average and normal. Occasionally, I experienced brief, insightful moments where I felt that there might be something special about me or I might have some innate greatness that would someday be known to everyone, but most of the time my reality was that nothing about me or the world I lived in stood out as exceptional. I was the third of four children, and while I was the only girl, I did not consider my gender to be a desirable uniqueness but rather an obstacle that would somehow limit me in life. I tried hard to be like my brothers. Often, I was labeled a "tomboy" because of my athletic abilities, the way I preferred to dress, or my somewhat competitive nature.

So there I was, an average kid living an average life, until one day at age seven something happened to change my life forever.

While it was unusual for my parents to leave us kids in the house with a young babysitter, they had to attend a back-to-school conference one evening, and they left a twelve-year-old boy in charge. I think my parents recognized something about him that was less than trustworthy; but still, that particular night they entrusted the care of me and my siblings to him.

As soon as my parents were out the door, the four of us decided to take advantage of our unsupervised freedom to engage in one of our favorite roughhousing games, one that we liked to call "train wreck." We all knew this was a game that our parents did not allow us to play because of the potential for injury and the likelihood of damage to the household furniture, but we were kids and the game was fun. So, one by one, from the oldest to the youngest, we raced through the kitchen like the cars of a train, then chugged into the living room at full speed. Over the top of a high-backed red couch we barreled and then landed completely laid out flat on the seat cushions, crumpling into the kids who flew before us—just like a train wreck.

When we had all landed, we would do it all over again. During one of the runs that evening, though, my upper lip collided with the elbow of my oldest brother. As the blood began to flow from my mouth, so did the tears. The babysitter took charge and instructed my brothers to settle down while he took me to the bathroom to tend to my wound. At first he was quite tender, preparing a cool, wet washcloth for me to wipe away the tears and the blood. But as my sobbing subsided he closed the bathroom door and ordered me to remove my clothes. Before we left that room, I had been stripped naked, forced to the floor, and raped.

Everything became surreal in that moment. I was floating above the scene watching and telling myself, "This isn't really happening to me." I was fighting to leave my body, but I could still feel the pain rhythmically cutting into my head and a sting that I couldn't explain between my legs. All of the emotional pain seemed to congregate in the swelling of my bruised lip, and I bit down hard to keep from screaming out.

When he was done with me, I was handed the same cold washcloth and instructed to clean myself up, get dressed, and keep quiet. The threats for breaking silence were more frightening than what had just happened to me, so I made the promise to him and to myself that I would never tell anyone.

Now I felt unique. I was sure that this had never happened to anyone else. Everything inside of me wanted to scream out, "This is not right!" but I took the vow of silence like a dedicated monk and walked out of the bathroom pretending that nothing had happened.

For weeks I walked around in a daze, hoping someone would notice that something about me was different, while at the same time praying that they wouldn't notice the immense shame I wore like a heavy coat. When the shock of what had happened finally wore off, I distinctly remember a moment of clarity that occurred while I was walking to school one morning. I had an inner knowing that this traumatic experience was one that would have a profound impact on my whole life. I also knew that as long as I kept the vow of silence, there would be no way for me to completely heal. I remember promising myself that I would never forget what happened, even though I had to push the memory to some part of my brain where it would not keep playing over and over. I also promised myself that someday I would find a way to heal the deep wounds.

That was the first time I was sexually assaulted. There were more occurrences over the next four years and several other perpetrators. It wasn't until I was twelve years of age that I broke the vow of silence and the scream finally came out. When I finally did speak the truth about what had been happening to me, I felt as though it was a turning point in my life, that the healing could actually begin. But by that time, I had already skillfully developed some extremely creative strategies for surviving in the world, and some habitual behaviors that were triggered by anything emotionally stressful. One of the most effective strategies that I became quite masterful at was dissociating. I could "check out," narcotize, leave my body or just reside in a fantasy land within my mind for days on end. As I grew older, these strategies became more sophisticated, and I felt as though I was leading multiple, contradictory lives.

Recognizing at age twelve that I had the potential to completely self-destruct with the unhealthy behaviors I was already trying, I found a way to police myself by joining a strict fundamentalist church. I devoted myself to the church and their rules in exchange for the safety net they provided. I had a place to go where I would not be molested, and people who held me accountable to their code of conduct. While this church was my home for a number of years, and I am truly thankful that I had a place of refuge, the moment that I challenged their rules, this family disowned me. I was excommunicated when I chose to date and eventually marry a man who was not a member of the congregation.

I felt as though I was free-falling, and my whole world was collapsing around me. I was back out in the cold, cruel world, all alone. Every belief I held about God and the Universe was snatched away like an umbrella caught in a mighty wind gust.

I attempted to rebuild my spiritual life only to find I had no mentors, no guidance, no beliefs of my own that I could call Truth. In fact, I had never really had a spiritual life, only rules and fear. In this place of emptiness, the wounds from my childhood began to bleed again, reminding me that I had promised myself healing someday. I enmeshed myself in my marriage, projecting all of the anguish I felt onto the partner I supposedly loved.

The marriage lasted seven painful years. It finally ended when my partner, who was in part the reason for my excommunication from the church, converted and joined the exact church I had been kicked out of. The irony is uncanny. I tried to return to the church with him, but by then I had begun exploring the world of metaphysics and realized at least one spiritual truth for myself, which was that my healing path did not lie in other people's dogma and rules. We parted ways, and I became the single parent of a five-year-old son, whom I acknowledge now as being one of my greatest teachers and healers.

It was at this juncture in my life that I began traditional psychotherapy to address the sexual abuse issue. In short, I was in and out of therapy for almost eight years, and while

I felt there was progress, nothing seemed to get to the core pain. I was able to intellectualize all of the healing tools that were handed to me. I took a certain amount of pride in mastering these tools, but I was still having nightmares and flashbacks of the abuse. My relationships with my family of origin were strained to say the least, and I could not bring myself to be in the same town, much less the same room, with my oldest brother, so I opted out of many family functions.

My behaviors became more and more contradictory, and my intimate relationships were completely dysfunctional. I began acting out sexually while at the same time experiencing sexual blocks that kept me from being intimate with anyone. The dissociative behaviors were in full swing, and when I couldn't check out on my own, I would self-medicate with painkillers, alcohol and/or marijuana. On the occasions that I didn't have access to drugs, I resorted to cutting myself just to get the sensation that kicked in when physical pain registered and opiate-like endorphins were released into my body.

On the flip side of all of this self-destructive behavior, the other life I was leading was that of a responsible, loving parent and full-time college student earning straight A's in a rigorous science program. Upon graduating college with honors, I opened a business and devoted myself to the hard work of being an entrepreneur and well-known leader in our community. Everything on the surface gave the appearance that I was a highly functional person.

Eventually, even my absorption with overachieving strategies was not enough to keep the monster in the closet. I knew on the deepest level that everything I was doing was part of an avoidance game, even the activities that appeared healthy on the surface. I also knew I had not kept the promise of healing that I had made to my seven-year-old self.

At the point right before I was introduced to The Journey, I felt as though I was the lone survivor of a horrific train wreck called my life. It wasn't a kids' game anymore. And yet I knew that everything that was happening was a culmination of that one game of "train wreck" I played as a kid and the pain that was never healed. I was stumbling around in a traumatic daze, shocked by the aftermath of destruction that surrounded me. I had destroyed an eleven-year relationship by having an affair; my once-successful business was on the verge of collapse, and I was meeting with bankruptcy attorneys; I was being sued by an upset client over some erroneous allegations and bleeding even more money to defense attorneys; my son was living on the streets at age sixteen, estranged from both me and his father, and dealing drugs; all of my so-called friends had abandoned me to side with my previous partner, who was the obvious victim of an unfaithful, cheating low-life; the woman I had had the affair with was about to dump me because she discovered that I had been lying to her about my ongoing drug use; and to top it off, I was being emotionally abused in that relationship but felt so alone and horrible about myself that I just rationalized it and told myself that I deserved it. I wasn't even a functional person anymore.

One evening as I sat in the darkness of my empty condo, I decided to write my farewell letter to the world. The pain was so intense, yet I had become so accustomed to numbing out, that all I could do was imagine the pain I must be in instead of actually feeling it in my body. Tears came, but somehow I still felt removed from them, as though they were not really mine but maybe those of a loved one who was looking in on the tragic train wreck, missing the beloved who never showed up at the train station. Still I wept, and once the tears began to flow, they kept coming. I wrote my good-byes to this life and all those I loved, and wept through the night and into the morning until exhaustion lulled me to sleep.

I awoke in the afternoon to the phone ringing, and on the other end of the call was the last person I expected to hear from, my then-tentative girlfriend, Lara. She invited me to meet her in the park for a picnic and lured me there with promises of peace between us. I pulled myself together enough to drive to the park, where we spread our blanket in the grass and sat in silence for a long time. Finally, she broke the silence and told me she had been to see a friend of ours who was also a therapist.

Guilt and defensiveness started to flood through me. I wanted to just get up and leave there and then, but there was some quality in the way she spoke that made me believe this conversation was not headed in the direction that I had expected. There was no story of, "You hurt me so much by lying that I had to go get professional help." In fact, there was no story at all. Instead, there was an invitation to open my heart and being to a new healing modality that she had experienced and that our friend was beginning to use in her practice.

She had brought a book with her called *The Journey,* and she asked if I would be willing to do a process with her from the back of the book. I was willing to do just about anything to get back into her good graces, so I agreed. I lay down on the blanket, closed my eyes, and she read to me the Emotional Journey process. I participated as much as I could, considering I knew nothing of how I was supposed to do this thing called an Emotional Journey. While I don't recall anything specific about the process itself, what happened afterward was nothing short of miraculous and was the event that spurred me on in my healing.

At the end of the process I opened my eyes, and Lara and I both just sat in silence again for what seemed like hours. As we sat there, my attention was drawn to a young man walking into the park about a hundred yards away from us. He had a peculiar energy about him, and he also appeared to be having a conversation with someone, but he was definitely alone. His pace was quite quick as he headed in our direction, and I could tell that he was so consumed with his ongoing dialogue that he did not even notice us sitting on our blanket in the grass, nor did he realize that we were right in line with the direction of his path. For several minutes we just watched as he drew closer and closer. His gestures were becoming more animated, and we started hearing the words he was speaking out loud. When I realized there was no cell phone in his possession, there was a moment of fear, and I questioned if we might be in danger, but neither Lara nor I moved or said a word as we continued to watch with wonder.

On some other-than-conscious level, the young man detected our presence and altered his bearing just enough to walk around us, but he did not acknowledge our existence in any way. Once he had passed, Lara and I looked at each other with a knowing sort of smile, like we had just barely skirted some peril.

And then he stopped dead in his tracks. He turned around and without coming any closer asked casually, as though there were nothing out of the ordinary occurring here, "May I ask you both a question?" We both nodded cautiously but curiously. "What would you do if you found out the person you love was smoking pot behind your back and then lying to you about it?"

This was just what I myself had done! How did this stranger know? I was stunned by the question he had just asked and the way he stood in front us genuinely awaiting an answer. It felt as though someone had just ripped open a freshly stitched wound, and the three of us were staring into the gaping hole, watching it bleed. He wore his pain in a way that for the first time made me understand how deeply my betrayal had hurt Lara. I don't recall the exact words that came out of my mouth or even what Lara said to him, but the essence of our response was pure compassion and forgiveness. I felt as though Lara for the first time really understood the pain that was underneath my choice to use drugs, and I understood the fear she felt when she considered losing me to an addiction. It was as though we were not really speaking to this young man but to each other. Then, after he heard what we had to say, he turned and kept on walking without any response.

In that moment, I remember feeling "truth bumps" all over my body. I had the thought that somewhere in the darkest moment of my life, grace had heard my cry and had sent this guardian angel to point the way home. I looked down at the blanket, and there was the *Journey* book staring back at me.

That same evening, Lara and I went to hear Skip Lackey, a presenter for The Journey in North America, give an introductory talk about The Journey at a local bookstore. We both knew within the first few minutes that we wanted to dive into the work. At the end of the evening I wrote a check for the upcoming weekend Intensive, draining the last money I had in my personal account. I had nothing to lose. When I got home that night, I folded my good-bye letter and placed it neatly in a drawer. I realized this would be my last attempt at healing this old, festering wound, and if I did not find any answers with The Journey, I surmised that the letter would be read by someone other than myself.

A few days later when the time came for the weekend seminar, I knew without any doubt that I had been guided to be there. This trust allowed me to relax, roll up my sleeves and let the processes have their way with me. In those two days, I discovered potent tools, a method for healing that would bring about lasting change in my life. In fact, they seemed to be the exact tools I had been praying for, because they worked on such a deep level, and the method was something I could use again and again. By the end of the weekend, I knew for the first time ever that there was a real possibility that I could finally fulfill the promise I had made to myself almost thirty-five years earlier. I could finally heal.

I was so moved at the end of the weekend by the healing that had already taken place for me that I decided to just dive in completely. I set a Monday appointment with one of the practitioners who had flown in as a trainer for the weekend. In fact, I booked the entire day with her to have an Abundance Journey process, draining the last money I had in my business account. Again, I felt I had nothing to lose.

There are very few processes that I've done over the last seven years since starting Journeywork that I remember in detail. Once an issue is cleared for me, it just seems to go, and the details of the process with it. But the Abundance process I did that day is one that I will likely never forget, because it shifted me and my life so profoundly. The process was designed to clear out blocks and limitations around abundance, and at its core it did exactly that, but it was also *the* process that finally fulfilled my promise to myself of healing. For the first time since being sexually assaulted at age seven, I was allowed to feel every emotion that I had pushed away, run from, numbed out, dissociated from or just ignored. The cellular release left me soaked in my own sweat and tears, and the forgiveness that came released me completely from my self-made prison. The healing that followed still seems miraculous to me, and while it is not the only process I've ever done around this issue, this particular one opened the door and set me free.

I began to see the effects of the healing immediately. I burned my good-bye letter and never considered it again. My business made a complete turnaround. Within eight months I went from being almost a half million dollars in debt to operating completely in the black and never having to file the bankruptcy. My marijuana and drug addiction fell away effortlessly, without any further intervention. My relationships began to heal, including the ones with my son, with my family and even with the people who had sexually abused me as a child. My relationship with Lara began to flourish, and all of the emotional abuse stopped immediately.

Lara and I have both deepened in our love and compassion for each other and continue to use The Journey Method within our relationship. We have manifested many wonderful things together: a beautiful home, healthy friendships and so much more, simply by clearing blocks and continuing to welcome every emotion as it shows up.

Over the last several years that I have been using The Journey Method, I have addressed the deepest, core issues in my life that used to keep me from living a joyous and authentic life. I can honestly say that I have been totally overhauled. What was once a train wreck is now a confident, integrated person who lives in the truth of what is here in each moment. I have access to all parts of me, which seem to be drawn from a bottomless well of talents, desires, dreams, emotions and greatness. The abundance that moves through me shows up in so many ways. I am particularly thrilled with the abundance of love that is my life and the ease with which creativity flows. I also have a newfound trust and willingness to follow my heart wherever it may call me to go.

Life is genuinely fun and meaningful, with a depth to it that I experience as simply lovely. When life happens, as it does, I know I have a set of tools in my belt that can help me through anything. And I know myself to be unique and special because we all are this, no matter what our story is.

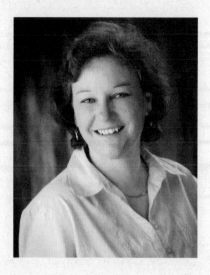

Lori Beaty *is an artist, entrepreneur, visionary, Conscious Coach and writer. She is passionate about cultivating creativity in herself and others using a wide array of integrated tools including Journey and Visionary Leadership processes, Non Personal Awareness (NPA), artistic awareness and development and shamanic healing practices. Lori is a regular presenter on Nightly Healing teleconference calls and is currently the president of Journey Outreach in North America. She offers both creativity and mandala workshops. Her coaching practice welcomes all who desire to flourish their creativity, heal creative blocks and raise their vibration through creative practices. You can follow her creativity coaching blog at www.clearlycreativecoaching .com or email her at lori@clearlycreativecoaching.com. You can also view her mandala art at www.collectivesourcemandalas.com.*

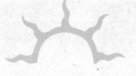

9

I Am a Rock

by Cynde Sawyer

Once upon a time, a long time ago (sixty-two years to be more or less exact), a woman wanted a baby. She had lost two daughters in life-threatening pregnancies and had a healthy son. But she wanted another child, so she lied to her husband and got pregnant. When those in her world found out about the pregnancy, her mother cried and beat on her son-in-law's chest, calling him a murderer. And the woman's husband, in fear, was very angry. The baby in the womb took it all in and made a vow to make the grandmother and father happy. And so a life of taking care of others and neglecting the self began.

The vow to please my grandmother was easy in that she was easy to love. She was the most important person in my childhood. I worshiped her and would do anything for her.

This was important, because when I was two years old I was angry at my brother, and picked up a block and threw it at him. My grandmother pointed her finger at me and said, "Girls don't do that." Wanting to please her, I made a vow not to do things that girls did not do. With limited knowledge of what that meant, I was left without a clear picture of how to be.

I could immediately see that girls did not feel anger (I extended that to not feeling anything at all), act on emotions or throw things. I did not know what to do with the anger, so I began a lifetime of suppressing it until it had to explode out of me. I lived a life of being very careful . . . holding on tight. This lasted until I was introduced to The Journey.

Although I did not realize it at the time, I was less than content in my life. My kids were grown, and my marriage became constricting—it did not fit me anymore. Things that *should have* made me happy did not. So instead, I told myself a story about being content, that nothing could really upset me. This heroine was strong and could handle whatever life threw at her. She lived each day by asking only to get through that day or that hour. She never needed nor asked for help. This story protected me from feeling what was really here. I was living in my story and carrying it around and showing everyone, "This is me, see me. Reward me for being my story." If asked, I would have said I really was content. It was a vanilla life, and I loved vanilla ice cream.

The cost was huge. Before The Journey, I was an extremely fearful person. Although my phobias were great, I was adjusted to this restrictive life. I planned everything in my life to avoid situations that would have brought up my fears. I was afraid of heights, so I never climbed anything. I avoided anything slightly high; even inclines of a parkway, curbs, stools or stepladders had to be carefully navigated. I taught my sons to aid me even in walking up and down stairs, calling it "gentlemanly."

I did not relish driving to new areas, fearful of unexpected bridges or highway entrance ramps. When I did find a bridge, I drove 15 to 20 miles per hour, fearful that I would lose control and fly over the side. I required that conversation in the car stop lest it distract me. Logically, of course, slowing down makes no sense; I was on the bridge even longer. However, I felt more in control. My sons were mortified by my bridge driving. My frequent trips to San Francisco required another driver, as I just held my breath while crossing the many bridges on route. Driving on the beautiful hills was a scary endeavor. Driving to new areas was fraught with problems. I had to figure out "routes of least fear." Mountains were out. Overpasses were bad, sometimes making me drive out of my way to avoid exiting the highway.

My fear of falling made it hard for me to fully play with my kids. I stayed in the background, baking, giving my kids the freedom to be messy and creative, rather than engaging in physical play. When my kids used playground equipment, I turned my back, too fearful to watch them.

My fear of heights stayed with me throughout my life— from growing up, into adulthood and to raising my children. Nothing eradicated it, not conventional therapy, not New Age self-growth seminars, not even the phobia cure we learned in an early seminar in the Journey Practitioner Program. This fear was bigger than a phobia. It dictated how I lived my life—or did not live it. It *was* my life; until . . .

I became aware of The Journey two years ago. I understand now that there was Guidance directing me to it. When a friend described The Journey to me and asked if I wanted to participate, "Yes" was loud and strong inside of me. And that first weekend Intensive affected me so greatly that I signed up for the program to become a practitioner.

Then, during the second and third full days of our week-long No Ego retreat, something very dramatic happened to me. It was both neurological and spiritual, and the most fearful moment of my life. I felt I was dying—not figuratively, but literally. I was left confused and hurting and terrified. Logic would have told me that that was not really happening, but logic was missing.

I did not "work through" this event; grace had other plans. At lunch break, I fled to my room to be alone and to "figure it out." It got worse. My emotions were so very big. I was crying and scared. I realized that being alone was not the right thing for me. I had lots of maneuvers and practice in suppressing feelings. I knew that if I stayed in my room, I would never leave to face this. Rather than push away the emotions, I left the room, went crying down the halls, and got help with facing the feelings. And then . . .

After No Ego, my husband and I went to the Grand Canyon and Sedona, Arizona. And suddenly, while viewing the Grand Canyon, I found myself climbing on rocks trying to get a better picture. I had no intention to do this. I just did it. I was amazed and impressed. I leaned over the canyon to get that perfect picture. Then I was jumping off of the rocks I had climbed, with no thought of where to put my feet.

On to Sedona. And there, I climbed up in a Jeep—to sit in the back of it! In the past, I would have fought (and won) to sit in the shotgun seat where on this occasion a handicapped woman needed to sit. I would have felt I was more handicapped than she. I would have helped her climb up the back: "Would you like me to get something for you to stand on?" I would have pulled my energy around me tightly to make sure I got what I needed. At our destination, instead of staying by the Jeep, I climbed the rock formations and walked around the top. I climbed on rocks that were scattered on the top. I could not get high enough. Going down the formation, I walked as though on a flat plane. My husband even got worried; he had never seen me like this. He started telling me that I did not have enough practice walking on this to be safe. Boy, was he wrong. I was safe.

Two months later, I drove to San Francisco in a rented car. I drove first over the Bay Bridge—halfway across I was laughing! I was driving the speed limit and loving every moment. I went over the Golden Gate Bridge, and then driving north I asked grace for *more* bridges! There were lots. (One seemed to go straight up and straight down. I made it. I decided, though, not to ask for more . . . enough is enough!)

At Life Transformation Week, the final class in the program, we were in Tahoe. There was a mountain there to conquer, and I rode the tram that went over the valley. I looked out and laughed; then I walked all over the top of that mountain. I was not on the regular paths, but in the open, hard-to-walk-on areas. I was free.

The Journey has changed my physical health, too: I got rid of headaches that plagued me for years. I never felt they were a problem because I had bigger fish to fry (or complain about). I had thought that the headaches were caused by my neck position, so I had bought lots of different pillows. I had switched to a buckwheat pillow, which did not help, but made me feel that I was doing something. Some days the headaches were mild and would last just minutes, and some days they lasted all day. They came three to four days a week. I did not realize how bad they were until they were gone after that first Journey Intensive weekend.

I had also had irritable bowel syndrome (IBS) since I was eleven years old. I did not know that was what it was called until sometime in the 1990s. I just always had severe constipation and then severe diarrhea. That was very inconvenient: going out for a big dinner was chancy. I thought I was allergic to *something,* and it caused the diarrhea. I had been to lots of doctors who never found anything. It was embarrassing and debilitating. The bathroom was *my* room in the house because I spent so much time there. Then, in July of 2008, I did a Journey process where I understood that I had made a vow to be "just like" my grandmother, whom I adored. Unfortunately, she had stomach cancer, and after her stomach was removed, she had bowel problems for twenty-three years. I felt such freedom from releasing the vow and the problem it had caused. (And what freedom is here now, even in the telling! I don't think I would have written about this in this format two years ago. Now, when it can help someone, I no longer feel that "private" issues need to be kept private. It is just a story, and not who I am.)

So, speaking of "story," during that first Journey Intensive weekend, I realized that the "story" of *who I am* was not how I needed to define myself. This story started with the birth of my twins. Having twins is a joy . . . and a lot of work for the first two years. The boys were colicky and cried sixteen hours a day in stereo for the first nine months or so. I had a daughter who was almost two when they were born, and before I could catch my breath after the twins, I got pregnant with my fourth, a son. When he was born, he was unable to nurse because of a problem with his tongue. When we finally got him to nurse, we discovered he had life-threatening allergies and the worst eczema that the doctors had ever seen. He was in such severe, constant pain. So when he fell and broke his wrist, and when he pulled his nail out of his nail bed, he never cried—he could not differentiate between pain and no pain, because some sort of pain was all he knew.

His allergies got worse, and he was referred to a doctor who had done a National Institutes of Health study on food allergies and eczema. This doctor felt my son was the worst case he had seen, and told me that my son's hold on life was precarious. I made a vow then and there to keep my son alive no matter what. I prayed to God to make my son okay. I prayed to my dead mother to intercede and make my son okay. My mother-in-law, when she was dying, told me that *she* would do all *she* could from the other side to help my son. I believed her, sort of. And when the doctors thought my son had a genetic disorder that would have killed him (moved him from "may die" to "will die"), I called my ultra-religious cousin and asked her to have her rabbi pray for him. My rabbi did not think that there was a God who would make one child live because of prayer and not another. Could prayer work or not? I had to cover all bases.

Six weeks later we were told he did not have the genetic disorder. Did the prayer help?

Emotions were another thing that I did not understand until The Journey. I had prided myself on not being an emotional person. I was contained. I was content. I was not depressed and really had no highs. Highs were too energetic for me. I just wanted to live in calm and quiet. I was very even tempered. I could get angry, but I would swallow it down after a short time. I was not one to keep the anger up. I would move on. Friends admired my unemotional state: I was a pillar of calm. When things got really stressful, I would hibernate and retreat into my home and myself. A friend recently told me, "You just disappeared for years."

When the doctors told me that my son's life was under threat, I was very upset and was shaking with emotion. So, of course, I quickly calmed down and took care of what was next to deal with. My son needed me to take care of him. I was calm and did not embarrass myself nor the doctors or nurses with emotional outbursts. I was a model of what a good mother should be. And I paid the price: I also had many surgeries, and got sick, and of course had IBS that whole time. I was constantly aware of my body and monitoring it for problems.

I could not even read a book that would bring up lots of emotion. No Stephen King for me. And I did read. Reading the right types of books was escape from emotional reality. Reading kept me from feeling. When I could not sleep because emotions threatened to come up, I would read until I felt calm, until I was centered, until I could go on.

I took no risks, because taking risks meant having emotions. Gambling was not for me; it would get my adrenaline going. I said it was silly to waste money. I did not watch sports. That would certainly make me feel something; therefore sports were silly. What a waste of good time to watch a game.

Even when I was deliberately welcoming emotions in my Journeywork, dropping down through levels of feeling was a sham for me. I knew what the emotion was, yes, and I really did not feel it. I saw it. It was outside of me. The word for the emotion would come up in my mind: "Fear." "Anger." My Source (experience of the Infinite) was usually an *idea* of "Calm" or "Peace."

One day in a Journey process, someone took me down through levels of emotions, and when we came to "Nothing," she had me walk around in it. I loved it. It was my favorite place to be. Being in "Nothing" meant no emotions. None. No constrictive emotion, no expansive feelings. Just nothing. I wanted to live here. I had *tried* to live here. My theme song was Simon and Garfunkel's, "I Am a Rock," because a rock feels no pain. I did not want to feel happiness either. That took too much energy. It made me tired just thinking about it. Actually, I was tired all the time. It was hard to do much.

All of this was a colorless life. When I did not feel emotion I was safe. But what *is* "safe"? Is there really any safety in this life? Is that what we are truly seeking?

And then there were the other unseen forces driving me . . . It wasn't until much later that in continuing my Journeywork I began to see the power of the beliefs, vows and rules that, unknown to me, were governing my life.

The way I see beliefs is that they are the glasses we put on to see the world. Anything we see is distorted or colored by the "glasses" we wear, our filters. We cannot see otherwise than through the glasses. We also will only hang out with those who share our beliefs; we walk away from those who do not. We don't believe them. If they try to convince us that we are wrong, we know *they* are wrong, and we don't question that.

Positive affirmations don't work when we don't believe them; yet we may not even know that we don't believe them! And I have found also that if we have a belief, we have almost certainly made vows surrounding it, too. And then there are rules that follow from that. For example, if I believe that I am stupid, I will feel like I am stupid at doing *everything* I do. If I do something smart, I will discount it. And I will have rules about stupid people: for instance, stupid people don't succeed in math, so I will never be able to balance my checkbook. That belief will in turn create vows: there might be vows about never trying to figure out any math. It will grow.

The vow to please my grandmother, made in my mother's womb, did just that; it set up a pattern that it was hard to break or even to recognize. Then the vow made when I was two—that vow not to do things that girls did not do—added another layer, and also expanded to encompass most things in my life. I have now found many beliefs, vows and rules that have hampered me, and when I let them go, I have found freedom. The belief that girls cannot feel emotions or act on them was powerful. I also had a belief that I had to be rescued: I almost drowned in Lake Michigan when I was four, and my mother rescued me. I could not have done it on my own. This belief expanded to create powerlessness throughout my life.

Then, I had a belief that I was responsible for the happiness of others and therefore had to control every situation and person to make sure the outcome was what *I* saw as what they needed. This belief was formed while I was little; when my parents would be fighting, I felt I was responsible for making them stop fighting and be happy. I did this by crying loudly, trying to get them to hear me and stop. Letting go of this belief was extremely liberating, and even though I still see it pop up occasionally, I no longer *believe* it! I now know the truth is everyone is responsible for their own lives, their own happiness, sadness, depression or anger. I can love them *and* let them experience what they need to experience.

I also developed a belief when I was newly born and in an incubator. I was crying and the nurses were talking next to me and ignoring me. I was not seen nor heard. I spent my life trying to be seen and heard, sitting front-and-center wherever I was, speaking loudly and forcefully. When I released this belief, I was able to sit in the back or the side or middle. It was a new perspective for me.

Now I understand more how our beliefs weave themselves together to form our story, and that people live in stories. These stories are not who *they* are, any more than *I* am defined by the stories of my past. It just does not matter anymore. There is unbelievable freedom in understanding this.

I had always defined myself through the story of being "a mother of a child whose life was precarious" and the struggle I undertook to keep him alive. People admired me because I was so strong, so capable and so very noble to be able to do this. With false modesty I would say, "Anyone could do it," but knowing damn well not everyone could! Did I trust *anyone* to take care of my son? No! *I* was the only one who could do it right and keep him alive! Who would I be, if not the parent of a child who could die, the mother of four, the mother of twins? At the end of that first Journey Intensive, I left that story behind.

If we are not our stories, then what are we? At the Journey events, we are told to "put out a powerful prayer." What does this mean? Can this work? In the past two years of discovery and self-exploratory work, I truly believe, first, that there is a very active presence of God. Second, that this very active presence is involved in our lives. Third, that there are answers to prayers, and fourth, that we *are* this presence of God. We are made up of God, not just made in the image of God, we are made *from* God.

I see in my life and in the lives of my clients that those for whom God is present easily expand and move into a higher place of being. Is this just mind? For me, no, it is heart. It is a bigger knowing. It is the place from where healing comes. It is the place from which we grow and become one with all. Being in The Journey and using The Journey Method have helped me open into this spiritual place.

Today I feel. I find myself at odd times smiling. It surprises me: I am happy! How strange is that? And it is okay to feel *everything*. I ask myself, "What is here now?" and get an answer through an emotion. On my recent trip to India with Brandon and many other Journey practitioners, we spoke a lot of giving up our "story," because the story is not who we are. I really get that. I really, *really* get that. I am not the story of the mother with the four children. I am not the story of the events in this life. I am not the story of even my emotions. I can feel the emotions, and I do not live them. Nothing defines me. I am. No description. No adjectives. No adverbs. I am. Yet at an even deeper level there is no separate "I" . . . just this Freedom.

I never really understood the power of gratitude before I started this work. Sure, I was glad when my son was doing okay and that my other kids were okay. However, the deep feeling of gratitude that I now experience surpasses anything that I felt before. My heart swells with the feeling; it is so enormous. I am grateful for large things and also for the small things in my life. As I am grateful for the opportunity to tell you my story—the story that is no longer "my" story—the story that has led to this beautiful place where I am free to feel, to be healthy and to live my life NOW. The rock has dissolved, and I am Freedom.

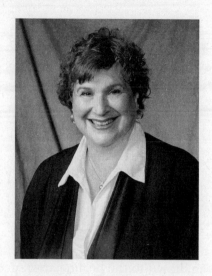

Cynde Sawyer *and her husband, Mike, live as empty-nesters in the Chicagoland area in a rural, peaceful setting; their children are now thriving as successful adults. Her hobby is ceramics, which gives her a creative outlet that she did not know she had earlier in life. Cynde has a passion to see people get beyond the beliefs that are holding them back from a life of freedom, happiness and love. She is an internationally Accredited Journey Practitioner personally trained by Brandon Bays, has been trained as an NLP Practitioner and is a Licensed Spiritual Health Coach. She integrates all the different processes to help clients gain freedom. Cynde can be reached via email at cynde@ thevisionaryway.com or at www.thevisionaryway.com.*

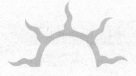

10

Cowgirl's Quest

by Robyn Johnston

I've always been drawn to the healing arts, specifically non-traditional forms of therapy. I was raised on a cattle ranch in North-Central Nebraska, so I didn't have a lot of support in this direction until my late twenties. Though my public school teaching career brought some pleasure and satisfaction, it wasn't real fulfillment. I felt empty, hollow inside. I knew that I wanted to do something different, so I began to explore.

My quest for spiritual truth led me down some pretty interesting paths. I discovered feng shui, the ancient art of placement. I became professionally certified and began to build a practice. From there, I began a deeper search for "Who I am" and "What I am here to do."

This need to know produced several interesting trips, trainings and experiences. One took me as far away as the Yucatán to learn a DNA activation process; another led me to Las Vegas, where I took a Despacho workshop with Elizabeth Jenkins. All this time I was working, being a wife and raising three adorable cherubs. Yet I was still empty inside.

By the end of 2007, I had had my fill. I didn't care if I ever went to another training again! Each experience was a valuable tool, but no teacher or training ever filled the gap that I felt inside. I felt resigned that "this is how it will be," and I stopped looking for teachers and courses to attend.

The following March, I received a call while waiting for a flight to Orlando with my husband and kids. It was my best friend, Ann. She started telling me about this great book she'd read and this program called The Journey that was going to be in Denver, and that we should take a girls' day and please would I consider going and oh yeah you have to register today . . . I told her that I had no intention of doing any more trainings, but when I heard the disappointment in her voice, I paused. She was my best friend after all, and sometimes she knows things! It would also mean spending time with her.

And so I relented. I called the Journey office, gave them my credit card number over the phone and booked for something called an Intensive, secretly dreading "another training." I hadn't even read the damn book . . . what was I thinking? Oh well, the plane was about to board, and I wouldn't have to worry about this for another month.

So, in April 2008, I ended up going with Ann and two other women to my first Journey Intensive. I consider this the day that I woke up. I don't say this lightly, as I had always thought that I had my life (and everyone in it) under control . . .

The first night I had an opportunity to put the day's revelations into practice. In a conversation with my husband, one where I would normally get sucked into guilt and drama for being gone, I simply didn't participate. Now, this may not sound like a novel idea, but for someone who's been raised to defend herself, have the last word and fight like hell for what she believes in . . . this was HUGE! I felt all the emotions in that conversation, and I let them be. I was flooded with anger, fear, resentment, gigantic guilt, a breaking heart . . . and more clarity and awareness than I'd ever had in the previous thirty-five years of my life.

I knew then there was something to this training that no other experience could hold a candle to. I didn't know what specifically, but I was intrigued and I was determined to find out more. Ann and I signed on for the next Journey workshop, the Manifest Abundance weekend. Again I tapped into some really deep stuff: some very, very old guilt and a lifetime of setting myself up for guilt came pulsating its way to the surface of my conscious awareness. I could no longer be blinded to the significant events of my life. There was no other person in the world to blame for holding me back—and the strangest thing was, I couldn't even blame myself!

After that weekend I went home and had a long talk with my husband and then my nine-, six-, and three-year-old daughters about completing the whole Journey Practitioner Program. I invited their thoughts and opinions and shared that I had some very important work to do for myself that would ultimately help me be a better person, wife and mommy. Two kids were for it, one against, and my husband simply said nothing. He'd been down this road too many times not to know that if he told me no, I would do it anyway; if he told me yes, I might think he was supporting me! After much contemplation, I knew that I wanted to continue with the program. I didn't *have* to, I *wanted* to. I didn't know how I was going to pay for the experience, I didn't know who was going to watch my kids, I didn't know where the forty-five case studies required for accreditation would come from. (I live in the middle of nowhere!) I didn't know how it was going to happen . . . I just knew that it would.

I dove into the additional modules, the countless processes, giving and receiving and each time gleaning more awareness. Life Transformation Week, the final week of the program, was a home run for me. For the first time in my life, I found what I was looking for—*me*. Each modality before this had peeled away enough layers that for the first time in my life I was able to see the "Who" of who I really am: the vastness that resides within and between these cells. Always before I'd been searching, wondering what title I needed, what role I was to play, and all the while hoping for a really big part. I'd tried my hand at so many things, and many of them just didn't work. When others around me were having significant breakthroughs and seeing themselves and their brilliant futures . . . I was seeing nothing. (Significantly, at the seminar I lost my name tag . . . three times! And what is amazingly cool is . . . I didn't mind.)

It seems like the crux of my life had been about fighting for recognition, acceptance and inclusion. I had done and said *anything* to become one of the "right people." I spent my early years pleasing my parents, and after that I went on to please my husband. I avoided conflict at all costs until I was backed up against a wall—but then watch out! I became an ass-kicking monster!

The point is that I had never stood up for myself because I was so busy worrying about hurting other people's feelings, much too worried about what others would think and say about me, while all the while pretending *I* had no feelings and emotions. Twisted, right? Yep, that was me. I had this vision of being a brilliant spiritual teacher, finding enlightenment and thus escaping the mundane aspects of my life. I'd taken umpteen million trainings looking for something to make me "loving, beautiful, peaceful, graceful, soft, elegant and wise." I laugh at this now, because the ego within this skin was searching for something that was already here, all the while denying true, authentic emotions. And while I was supposedly suppressing my anger, it was spewing in all directions . . . while my mind pretended to be a yoga-loving, meditation-inspired guru!

I hope that you can see that one of the most brilliant and treasured gifts that The Journey has helped me recover is humor and the ability to laugh at my own human-ness. I have a lot of fun at my own expense these days, as I realize I can be pretty brash, a bit crude and downright silly, and it's okay. I'm not trying to fit into a perfect mold anymore. I just take what's here and have fun with it.

The Journey has helped me to excavate parts of me that I didn't even know I liked. Each process is a stepping-stone back to my true identity, which is really a limitless blank canvas open to all possibility. This work has helped me release the need to cling to a role, an image or a part. I get to choose whatever part I am playing! If I don't like it, then I go to the screenplay within and make adjustments.

Prior to The Journey, I was a scary, control-freak mom. I had come close to losing my middle child twice. Both episodes left me reeling and writhing in pain. During The Journey's No Ego retreat, these issues powered to the surface. I decided to fight Death with everything I had . . . and yet in my final process of the retreat, Death took *me*. I was surprised to find at the end of the process that I was still here—and then I realized this "I" was no longer the "I" that I had known.

It took me a while to figure this one out. (Parts of me are probably still trying to make it all compute, and that's okay.) This was one of the most terrifying experiences I've ever had, but one of the most transformational. I came back to my daily life knowing that it's not me that pulls any strings, and I can't function as puppet master in my life. This awareness has served as a significant source of solace in times when old habits of worry have arisen. My mind doesn't go on walkabouts in this direction anymore, because my Being instantly starts questioning the "What if's." I think moms are programmed to be protective, to worry and to fear for their children, though The Journey has helped me see that such fear is a detriment most of the time. It isn't the kids, it is *me* that is miserable! I am so grateful that I have The Journey Method to assist as my children enter the teen years. I have a feeling I'll need that support!

I could go on and on, sharing many revelations and insights; that would be denying the real reason that grace has tapped me on the shoulder to share my story. My heart is pounding now, even as I type, because what you are about to read is the raw truth of what The Journey actually did for me.

As I said, my past pattern was to avoid conflict and judgment. I would stop at literally nothing to prevent anyone from knowing anything "bad" about me. I hid behind that "good girl" façade so that I wouldn't have to experience shame or guilt or judgment. I was young and immature at the time and didn't have the awareness about life that I do now, so there is no blame, only compassion for the younger me. I honestly have to say, though, that I never thought I'd be sharing this story with anyone else . . . ever.

When I was nineteen, I was in a relationship with a young man whom I dearly enjoyed being with. My parents and only brother hated him. So you can imagine when I became pregnant that there was little support, a whole lot of judgment and even more guilt. My parents were heartbroken, and so was I. I had a tough choice to make, and of course, I was one of those persons who had said, "That will never happen to me . . ." Yep, never say never.

I remember sitting in my dorm room crying. Not because I wanted to keep this baby, either. I was crying because I didn't want my perfect image to be destroyed. I was from a small town. Small towns can be brutal, especially if you do anything wrong. I went from being at the bottom of my class to salutatorian (not *that* big of a deal, there were only twelve kids!). My parents had never had a shot at higher education because I came along when my mom was seventeen. So I had worked hard, gotten great scholarships and was going to be *the* girl in my family to have graduated with a degree from a four-year college.

I buckled to the pressure; I could not have this baby. I couldn't let my folks down, and I couldn't stand the humiliation, talk, judgment, criticism and all that pain that would come with getting "knocked up." I just couldn't do it. I'd love to say that I wanted to have the baby and that I wanted to marry this guy, but that wouldn't be the truth. In fact, I didn't even know the truth, or what steps I would take to find it. I was so used to doing *everything* that my parents or anyone else told me that I literally would *not* make a decision that invited any kind of judgment.

It wasn't until much later, through a Life's Purpose Journey process, that I discovered that I'd been pleasing people my whole life. I'd been set up from an early age to do so, and by age nineteen, I was set on my course of pleasing people no matter what the cost. My life continually created lessons where I would have to compromise, swallow and deny my own truth. I was stuffed to the gills with no way to let it out. In fact, I was searching for anything but the truth . . . because, to my perception, the real truth of my past was too ugly. What spiritual teacher could admit that she did this horrible thing simply for reasons of vanity? That's sick.

In my Life's Purpose process those walls came down. Slowly the mortar turned to liquid tears, and slowly the crumbling happened. I wasn't forced to see anything ugly; I was led to an opening within my being. Peering through the portal, I saw the real truth of who I am. I had a conversation with the baby, this being who I "took the life from," and received the most amazing message that let me know everything was fine. All I can say is that a miraculous healing occurred, erasing self-destructive patterns, decades of guilt and most of all, the fear of finding and totally standing in my truth . . . *no matter* what others think.

I have a feeling there are others out there who have also compromised their truth to keep the peace, others who have denied their truth to keep those around them happy and comfortable. We do this, it's not a sin, we just do this.

How has this changed my life? When I opened into the reality of my actions, there wasn't the hell and damnation that I expected. Instead there was peace, and not just a little, either. I became so filled with light that for a time I had no need to eat or sleep. I feel I received healing at a level I can't put words to, healing that took a while to trickle back into my life stream in miraculous ways.

First, I was able to really stand in my truth with my mom. I've always felt compelled to make her happy and please her. This was ingrained from an early age. My mom is a loving, fiercely protective mother whom I adore, so I knew that these were *my* perceptions and it was time to work with them. I'd already released immeasurable fear, so pissing my mom off was the least of my worries! It happened, too. Shortly after my return from Life Transformation Week, the relationship with my mother hit a wall. This is probably what I had feared for years—and now it was happening and . . . I was okay with it! I stated my truth and discontinued contact with her for several months.

Though it may sound harsh, this needed to happen. I know without The Journey and the powerful process work available to me, I would never have had the strength to do this. I was healing a codependent pattern that had restricted me all my life. What has come through since then is a very healthy, clear relationship. My mother is fully aware of where I stand, what I support and what I am no longer willing to allow. We now talk weekly. We've reconnected on a new, healthy and mature level. What a blessing!

The other relationship that has shifted is the one with my husband. I was twenty-one when I got married. I went from being submissive with my mother to doing the same with my husband. I followed him around and did everything I could to please him and make him happy. I was a loving, supportive and spineless wife—and he liked it! I've tried to fit into a mold for him as well, being the perfect wife and perfect mother, doing and saying just the right things to keep the peace.

I really did try to be subtle when I came home from Life Transformation Week. This was a man who supported my constant searching for the truth and was pretty darn kind, even though I knew my search made him scared and miserable at times! I didn't want to shock him with my new awareness by "boldly speaking the truth." Actually, this may have scared him more, because he was used to me throwing a fit when I didn't get my way (a wonderful technique I picked up around age fourteen or so!). I think what shocked him the most after that week was that I didn't engage. When he dropped the "hook," I didn't bite. That's not saying I don't get mad, I still do. I am just aware of the triggers now. I think me finding my truth was one of the hardest shifts in our marriage, and I really can't fault him for it. He married me as I was then; he wasn't planning on my changing. And he loved me, all of me, even the parts that I kept hidden from myself.

When I started to get clear on what I liked and what I didn't, it was a big change. My husband's a cowboy, and he spends most of his time in the summer going to rodeos. I followed him around for fifteen years. Last summer I didn't. I didn't mind if *he* went, but *I* was not interested in living on the road anymore. I wanted to be a homebody. I wanted to play with the kids, go camping, grow a huge garden and hang out near the fire pit at night. He went his way and I went mine, and we stayed married.

Then he forgot my birthday, and I got mad. What a gift this was! In the past I would have stewed internally in my resentment for months; without that old pattern, I simply stated the truth, my deeply hurt feelings, and got on with my life.

I found a lot of things about our relationship that were no longer supportive. I sat with this fact for a long time. For years, I feared getting a divorce, living on my own, raising my kids, etc. Now I realized that my truth was just that: my truth, not his. I wanted certain things, and I was no longer willing to compromise. I shared what I needed most, what I was willing to work with and what I would do if he couldn't meet those needs. And then I let it go. I realized for the first time in my life that Truth was my partner; anyone on the outside was simply a reflection. I understood that my needs for love, affection and companionship were important enough for me to stand up for, even if it meant that I would offend, anger and run off the person I most wanted to receive them from. Only then did the distance in our relationship, created ultimately by my connecting with my own truth, become an amazing solace. I was willing to allow him time to accept this revelation, and if he couldn't, then I would move on. Either way, I was going to be happy!

Last December I chose to adopt a Shih Tzu. My husband doesn't like dogs in the house . . . at all. While I can respect his opinion, I am the one who cares for, cleans and organizes the space from floor to ceiling. I want a dog, and that is true for me! We've had many discussions about Marley, some very tense. I can comprehend and appreciate the fact that my husband doesn't like animals in the house, and I also know that I am fully living truth as it shows up for me. It may not look like *his* truth, and that is sometimes difficult. Remember, I've spent many years pleasing others, so while it may sound self-centered, selfish and immature, I will not back down! Call me strong-willed, call me stubborn, call me anything . . . it simply makes no difference. I *love* having an adorable gray furball, sitting right here at my feet as I type. Had I compromised my truth, I would not have had the rich experience of having a loving four-legged companion to share my life with.

And sometimes standing in my truth is no "walk in the park." I've continually had opportunities to deny and forget this reconnection with myself. In some cases, it probably would be easier to betray myself, but I've already learned that easier is not always the right way for me.

Being true to this Truth is what I live for every day, even if it doesn't make sense to anyone else. I find that I am much more willing to take risks; I am more brave, bold and daring. I don't go looking for something to "fix" or find ways to boldly express my opinion. In fact, I still tend to shy away from conflict if I can; yet after sitting for a while and letting truth resonate, when I need to, I will speak. I know that what I say is often not what others want to hear or what they expect to hear, but it's my wish that Truth will be expressed through my Being and theirs—not just my truth or their truth—but Truth.

It doesn't matter what *I* have to say. What matters is that Truth resonates within those who seek it. It took me some monumental lessons to figure that one out! I kind of like to think that grace had it all designed that way; that every event that happened wasn't good or bad, it was simply Truth that kept knocking on my heart's door. Truth didn't give up on me; it just kept finding ways to reveal itself. I am deeply grateful for The Journey because it became the key that allows Truth to open that door and keeps it wide open.

I had always wanted to be someone else, living in a hip location, doing healing work, driving a new car, living in a beautiful home, having it all. Now I've come home. It doesn't look anything like the image my mind/ego was conjuring up. It's pretty basic, very down-to-earth and nothing flashy. However, there is a spring in my step that wasn't here before. Instead of loathing living in the country, far away from Whole Foods, I'm discovering an entirely new adventure—growing my own organic foods. I am excited about the future, though I have no idea what it will look like when it becomes the present.

I am letting go of a lot of debris, physically, mentally and emotionally. I don't know if I will ever have a big office with lots of clients. I don't know if I will ever get the chance to speak to crowds of people and share my story with them. I don't know if anyone other than my husband, kids and dogs will ever see the zest for life that I've found and the joy that resonates for just being me! I simply welcome the healing that can come through my being because this time around I know "I" am not the one doing it! If people see me as beautiful, successful, happy and prosperous, it is because all that already exists within *them*. And if they see something other

than that, perhaps it is Truth that is patiently, gently knocking on their heart's door.

Those who experience and live The Journey know that
when we commit to this work we are sometimes surprised
by the outcome. Very recently I was blessed with such an
unexpected gift. Remember the young man I wrote about?
I haven't had contact with him in nearly seventeen years.
Then out of the blue I got a Facebook friend request from
him! I was very shocked and did a mini-process right there
in front of my computer! Whew. After some light conversation and comments back and forth, I sent a message stating
that I never meant to hurt him. I simply said, "I hope that
you were able to find peace and healing." Within a week's
time, we were able to chat by phone, and of course I mentioned The Journey and my experience thus far. I sit here
in the awe of grace-filled bliss. I am sending him a *Journey*
book and have offered to assist him in finding wonderful
practitioners to work with if he so chooses!

It wasn't The Journey that *did* anything to me. It was
grace working through The Journey that helped my soul
find what it's always looked for . . . TRUTH. I heard Brandon continually say, "Call off the search." I am happy to report that it is forever on hold. Why would I need to look
anywhere else to find what I've been looking for my whole
life: ME? To find the Being who resides in this cellular
house, the Being which is pure spirit, grace, bliss, peace,
beauty, light, laughter, hope, joy? For that I am grateful beyond words. The doors of my heart are wide open, and it's
my prayer that they stay that way.

I'm not perfect at the human level, and now I'm not try-ing to be. I embrace the totality of my being on all levels and am deeply grateful for the opportunity to incarnate into such rich experience.

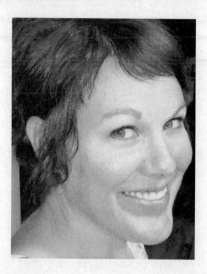

Robyn Rae Johnston *is a Nebraska cowgirl who enjoys wearing a variety of "hats" such as Accredited Journey Practitioner, Licensed Spiritual Health Coach, Professional Feng Shui Consultant and li-brarian. Robyn's joy in life and her ability to help others see new perspectives are shared through her writing, teaching, speaking and personal sessions. When not riding her horse, tending a garden or gathering eggs, Robyn loves spending time with her family hiking, biking, camping or golfing (basically anything to be outside!). She can be reached via email at cre8tivecowgirl@gmail.com. Her website is www.open2awareness.com.*

11

On the Wings of a Prayer

by Kimberly and Arsene Tootoosis

KIMBERLY:

We met in 1978, my husband Arsene and I. I feel grace/ God spoke to us from our first moment together. I feel the guidance was present from the beginning and through all the challenges of growing together, and especially coming to know ourselves and our own paths in this life. We had similar interests, similar goals and a deep vision and commitment to serve and help others. This common ground seemed to allow us to face many unforeseen challenges and be able to overcome them. And with such good intent, and living as healthily and positively as we were able, we never expected the health crisis Arsene was to face in 2003.

I chose to marry and raise our four children in the community of Poundmaker, feeling it would connect them to the earth and the strong spiritual and cultural way of life of the Cree and Nakoda people. I knew this to be certain in my heart: that they naturally would set deep roots down and still have the ability to fly and experience the world. After raising my children and doing the best I could the best way I knew how, I felt the diagnosis of myelodysplasia (also defined as smoldering leukemia) that my husband was given was not only going to be a challenge, but that it was also going to provide us with our greatest teaching. In that understanding, in seeking spiritual help and guidance in our lodges, it was said time and time again that Creator and the grandfathers hear our cries and help us and that we too needed to do our part.

After thirty-three years of coming home to this way of life, I finally truly understood to the fullest extent what that statement meant. I remember my youngest son Mylan telling me one day after countless ceremonial doctorings my husband had endured, "Mom! We can go to the wisest elder, the most powerful medicine man, find the strongest medicine, go to the ends of the world seeking prayer, but if God decides to take Dad or decides He has another purpose for him or needs him . . . He will take him. All we can do is ask, Mom, ask that He pities us and lets Dad stay longer with us, that He lets him stay and do His work for Him here."

That night in the lodge, in my deepest prayer I asked for help; that we be shown what was next in our healing. I knew that our crisis had a purpose, a deep purpose, and it was coming to teach us, as most challenging and painful experiences do.

Not long after that, Arsene and I were browsing through a bookstore. I had long since stopped spending too much time with self-help books, having found many repetitive. On this day, as I walked through the aisle, my eyes fell upon a particular book that drew me back down the aisle twice to glance at it. This is where the expression "the book literally fell off the shelf into my hand" rings true for me. Handing the book to Arsene, I said, "I think you are to read this"—knowing also deep in my heart it was meant for me as well. I actually completed the book, *The Journey*, by Brandon Bays, before he did, having picked it up every time he put it down.

Thus began our experience with The Journey.

ARSENE:

During our life together, Kimberly and I have had a deep intent and commitment to each other, to our family and to helping others, primarily our Indigenous people. Our family has always moved forward quickly to seek a path of wellness and healing. Recognizing in later years our similarity in childhood experiences and traumas, as well as the generational impact of historical traumas, we focused hard on our studies and our careers, with an emphasis on the healing and wellness of our families and communities. We did our best to work effectively together and to facilitate and encourage positive, healthy lifestyles for ourselves and for the people we worked with.

Our greatest source of strength and the roots of our foundation is our cultural and traditional lifestyle, a life of ceremony, prayer, song and dance. Although maintaining a well-balanced lifestyle can be challenging in any society, it was especially so with ours. We were determined to keep moving forward no matter what, overcoming our own challenges in parenting and in our relationship.

Little did we know that the biggest challenge of all was at hand: my diagnosis with myelodysplasia. It stopped us in our tracks. The news was devastating for me and my family. Now what? It took all we had to keep it together and face our fears, our challenge. "Smoldering leukemia" are scary words, and the idea of a stem cell transplant as the recommended treatment, and the need for a bone marrow donor, was overwhelming. In the midst of this, I felt drained and completely overwhelmed, mentally and emotionally. My energy level was dropping almost daily as I got weaker and weaker.

As I acknowledged the emotional waves, I felt anger which became a deep rage, and added to that was a deeper fear. I was angry at everyone. I blamed everyone and everything under the sun for my getting sick. I blamed God because I was angry at God. I wondered why this was happening when I had made strong commitments to serve what was good and positive in our life. I was living in a good way and following the spiritual teachings in my family. Why was this happening?

I soon realized this attitude was not doing any good. I needed to make a choice: to want to live—or to give up and die. As soon as the reality entered my mind that "I can die from this disease," I chose to live. I put out the deepest prayer ever, whispered from my heart and soul, and I cried for help. I spoke to God.

I recall in our ceremony praying and saying to myself, "I will get well! I will recover! Whatever it takes, whatever way, wherever it is, I will find it or it will find me. Please guide us and tell me what it is I must do or what it is I am not doing." My faith has never faltered through my life, and again I felt determination to move forward and focus on what was present in my life. I refused to quit. I continued working, and I continued with the blood transfusions during the nine months prior to the stem cell transplant. A blessing is that our work involves group work, and it was a godsend to have people present throughout our work that understood my need to slip out for few moments. As Kimberly worked with the group, I would go and take a nap, as my energy level was dropping daily. Still I would always return to the group and to the energy that I needed. I danced right up to the last fall celebration, even though I was tired. I wanted to be in the healing energy of our people at the powwow celebrations.

A month before the transplant, Kimberly came upon the book *The Journey* in a local bookstore. She skimmed through it and asked me to check it out. I did, and after reviewing it, I decided to purchase it. It was interesting to watch Kimberly pick the book up each time I put it down, and soon she had it finished even before I did. She later told me about the experience of being drawn to that book, which is unusual, as she felt she had her fill of self-help books over the years. I had noticed her returning to this particular book a

number of times while we were in the bookstore. I believe
she is one who can verify the statement, "the book literally
jumped off the shelf and fell into my hands!" I found it interesting indeed, and smiled when she spoke those exact
words during a presentation in one of our groups describ-
ing The Journey and our experience in finding this process
work.

When I finished reading the book, I sat in silence and
in awe. I was alone, and I felt a peace and a calming that
was so deeply present. My thought was, if Brandon can recover from her health challenge, so can I! I was so amazed
at how profound Brandon's experience was. I appreciated
her honesty and her openness to share her own truths. I was
drawn into and became a part of her story in a way I cannot
describe. I felt very present as I turned each page. As I sat
there in that moment and placed the book down, I simply
knew in my heart that this was part of my prayer unfolding. It was up to me to use the tools presented. The gift was
in knowing that we picked up the book for that reason and
that reason alone.

Kimberly called the Journey office at the number listed
in the back of the book. She reached Kristine, who we later
found out was the wife of Skip Lackey, presenter of The
Journey in the United States. There was an Accredited Journey Practitioner in Calgary, Alberta, who was the closest to
us, and I decided to fly there to experience my first Journey process. Arriving back the same day, I asked Kimberly
to call Kristine once again to find out where and when the
next Journey seminar was. We decided we would invest

what we could and take the trip down to the States. Within a couple of weeks we were driving to Boulder, Colorado, to participate in a Journey Intensive workshop.

Having experienced many healing workshops, modalities and approaches, we made the decision to put all our expectations and ideas aside. We were to attend this workshop solely for ourselves, completely immerse ourselves in the experience and place aside all our own preconceived ideas. At the same time, we would be cautious: we had always been careful in the previous years, strictly reviewing and evaluating countless approaches and models that are used with the healing and recovery process of our Indigenous people. Having encountered some unhealthy approaches and violent therapies, I was one to be vigilant about the credentials, evaluations and expertise of people working in our First Nation communities.

I wish to share a very intimate moment that I hold near and dear to me. As people, we all experience many sacred moments in our life, and the more open we are, the more those moments unfold for us. Sometimes they appear or unfold in ways we do not expect. When we arrived at the workshop, Kimberly and I both chose to sit in the front row, directly in front of the presenter. After all, we were attending completely open-minded and prepared to experience this wholeheartedly. On the second day, again seated front and center, a moment in the presentation had us sitting quietly and meditating while a most beautiful song was played. I recall hearing the beginning of the song clearly—and in a moment it slipped away. In its place was a most familiar and sacred song I hold close to me. I heard it so clearly and precisely, and stayed fully present with it. At the end of the song, I turned to Kimberly and asked if she heard the singing as well. She did not! Again it was revealed to me that I was on my own healing journey, and I was exactly where I needed to be. I also felt and knew in that moment I was going to recover. I was going to live. It was not my time to leave.

Our first Journey Intensive was a powerful experience. We found it at a critical time in our life, and I feel it came on the wings of my prayer. Those who have faced critical incidents in life will understand that sometimes we are in situations where we can only hope and pray and totally trust in Creator no matter the outcome. I had renewed hope, and though I was at my weakest physically, I felt stronger and more determined than ever.

Before leaving the group in Boulder, we approached Skip Lackey and Kristine and asked how we could secure the workshop in Saskatoon, Saskatchewan—Saskatoon being the central point of the province. Because The Journey Method stimulates healing at the cellular level and can also clear generational traumas and memory, and having experienced it ourselves, we saw the value of the process work as a tool in the healing and wellness of our people. We learned that the workshop was able to come to our area as long as we had enough support from people in the area willing to experience a Journey Intensive. We began sharing the information and the work with our children, our families, our clients and groups we worked with. The first Saskatoon

Journey Intensive was held the following fall. First, though, we invited many of our people to attend an Intensive in Edmonton, Alberta, so that we would have a sufficient number of workshop "graduates" as trainers to support the Intensive in Saskatoon. As a result, I recall the first Journey Intensive in Saskatoon as being approximately 90 percent First Nation as well as attracting great interest and a large number of participants.

The month after our trip to Boulder, I went through my stem cell transplant without any complications. My recovery was speedy, and I recall my doctors asking me what I was doing to be recovering so quickly and with minimal discomfort. I stated that daily prayer, my spirituality and way of life, as well as the Journey process work, were what helped me the most. I continued doing the Emotional and Physical Journey processes and attending a Journey Intensive whenever possible. My doctors also requested to enter my story into their medical journal, recounting my progress. It was part of a research study, and they wanted to know what was helping me recover quickly with very few or none of the complications that I was forewarned about.

I know in my heart and in my actual experience that our ceremonies and the Journeywork fully complement each other. I continue to live fully and embrace this way of life and the tools I have that help me. I attend the Intensives that we have secured in Saskatoon every six months. I continue with my self-care daily. And I work with others. It is great to see people dive into the process work and find forgiveness and freedom in whatever issues are present for them.

I feel that any healing process is successful if and only if an individual lets go and trusts the process, letting all judgment and limiting beliefs fall to the side. I faced my fears and doubts and overcame them.

Spirit is alive. We can connect to that Source inside us and thrive from that place. Our spirit as a people was never destroyed. Spirit cannot be destroyed. I am alive and well until Creator decides.

Life is awesome.

Thank you, Creator and grandfathers . . . A-ho.

Thank you to my biggest support, my beautiful wife, Kimberly, my children, my family. Thank you, Edwin and Milly, Skip and Kristine Lackey, Brandon Bays, Kevin Billett and Arnold Timmerman and the whole Journey family, and the countless friends and family who have walked with us in our work. Thank you, thank you, thank you.

KIMBERLY AGAIN:

I work now at a much deeper level and walk beside people healing at this level and in the reconnection to Spirit, Spirit that was never wounded. Spirit cannot be destroyed or damaged. It is up to each of us to reconnect and live from that place completely and truthfully. I give thanks every day for life and for love. I give thanks for the guidance and for having the spiritual way of life that we do. I am grateful my children were born and welcomed into a powerful circle of life and were completely immersed in such a blessed way of living. I see how it has allowed them to grow and learn and see the gift of life. I have witnessed them diving into the Journey process work and sharing it with others. I am grateful for the Journey family worldwide that supports and encourages them. I can see worldwide healing unfolding. I have seen how this most unique and dynamic process has been welcomed into the Indigenous communities of the world. I am grateful for the healing I have experienced and most grateful that Arsene continues to walk beside us.

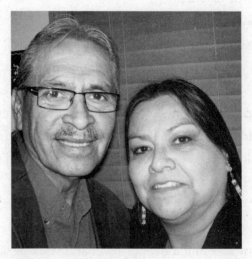

Arsene and Kimberly Tootoosis *are both founders of Red Echo Associates and work together as therapists and trainers. They provide workshops and trainings to First Nation/Indigenous communities and have worked in the field of healing and wellness since 1983. They can be reached at 306-398-4746 or 306-441-0725.*

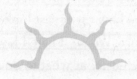

12

The Decision

by Susan D'Agostino

I could not believe what I was being told. There was no doubt in my mind—until this moment—that it *wasn't* cancer. The surgeon went on to tell me when my surgery was scheduled, and all I could hear was someone in the far distance talking; saying things I couldn't hear because my heart was beating so loudly in my ears. I was beyond shocked; I was in a different dimension.

Shortly afterward I lay down on the operating table, seemingly without choice: a cancerous tumor called invasive ductal carcinoma grade 2, estrogen positive, progesterone positive, was growing in my right breast. I was cut open . . . mutilated . . . a piece of me carved out of my body. Afterward, I felt numb, staring at the stitches that kept my breast from coming apart. My eyes stung with tears at the full realization of how weak and violated I was.

Of any part of my body I would have reduced, my breasts weren't on that list. Having my perfect breasts reduced to less than perfect made me doubt myself. Was having surgery the right choice? Had it been my decision? Did I have any other choice? I hated how my breast looked. It didn't feel like a part of me anymore. Worse, I hated how I felt, and I hated that I didn't have a clue about what to do to *not* feel this way.

My husband's friend told me breast cancer on the right side means anger and resentment. Who was *he* to tell me that? It was none of his business; he didn't even *know* me. He couldn't have known how anger lived at the center of my being, the demon inside I tried so hard to keep secret. *It* lashed out at my husband. *It* kept me in a constant state of irritability. After years of attempting to rid myself of this negative emotion, anger still had control of me.

It was a hot Saturday afternoon in the middle of summer, and I lay in bed crying. I felt weak, in the depths of despair, waiting for the doom of chemo and radiation. Fear at the thought of these treatments sucked the energy out of my body and terrorized my mind. I didn't want to be sick . . . to lose my hair . . . to have poison injected into my veins. I was terrified it would kill me. I didn't know what to do. I didn't know anything. *I didn't know anything!* I picked up the phone and spoke to someone who had done natural therapy. She advised me about some avenues I could explore and spoke of the alternative therapies that were available. She also told me to get passionate about life. I honestly didn't know how to get passionate about life but, suddenly, I knew something: *I wanted to live!* Relief spread through my body. I could feel *hope*. After hanging up the phone, I bounded out of bed, got into the shower and headed for the organic farm for some fresh vegetables to juice.

Mainstream or alternative? A decision had to be made. Sitting alone in our family room, engulfed by mind-numbing indecision, I felt the fear pulling at my insides. How do I decide what to do? What if I made the wrong choice? Then I had a powerful recognition that my body felt strong when I thought of alternative therapies but weak when I thought of chemo and radiation. A strange inner knowing came over me that if I listened to my body, it *would* guide me. It felt right. More than that, it felt like trusting my body's wisdom could be the best thing that ever happened to me. That is the decision I made: to build my immune system instead of destroying it.

The first three naturopaths I met said they couldn't help me, because of the stage and type of cancer I had. I was devastated but remained determined. Then I did find a naturopath whom I was comfortable with and who could help. I also discovered some other healing modalities that resonated with me and that could work in conjunction with naturopathy. I had found my healing path.

Exhaustion was a constant companion as I finished my treatments of high doses of intravenous vitamin C. Knowing I was going back to work in a couple of months didn't help any and caused me a great deal of anxiety. The truth was, I hadn't liked my job for a good many years.

After reading a few books on the law of attraction, I began to realize that maybe I *could* have the life I always wanted. Although, in truth, I didn't have a clue what that life would be like, because I hadn't dreamed of or wished for anything in such a long time. I decided to quit my job. I didn't know if it was the right decision, but it was *my* decision.

Little did I know this was only the beginning of the healing process; the body, the physical, was only the first component on the way to wholeness. Next came the spirit, the mind and the emotional parts, all wanting some attention and tender loving care. I took long walks in the forest that was close by my home and was mesmerized by its beauty. The magnificent trees seemed to calm my fears and doubts about whether I was healed or not. Some days I walked along the beach. Soon I began to experience insights about my own life as well as my friends' lives; it was as if this knowledge was there to be known by anyone accepting of it. I asked and prayed to my angels and guides daily that I would release the negative thoughts and feelings from my mind and body.

Some days, though, all I could muster up was, "Help me, help me, help me!" The fear, doubt and annoyance I felt toward my husband was overwhelming at times, so all-consuming that I thought for sure I would never get past it. He had begun a home renovation just before my diagnosis, and it was beyond my capacity to tolerate the mess and the constant arguing about what really needed to be done and what didn't. He does amazing work, that wasn't the issue; the problem was the length of time it was taking and the fact that he didn't complete one project before starting another one. When, in the family room, there were bare two-by-fours and a plywood floor, and that was left while he changed the windows in the opposite part of the house, it was maddening to say the least. From my perspective, it was as if he liked to see just how bad the house could look, and how much he could aggravate me and feed the constant fear and anger that kept showing its ugly head. Communication had never been our relationship's strong point, so it felt like nothing was in my control anymore as *he* did what he wanted, always disregarding anything *I* said.

When I told him I wanted a divorce, that just added fuel to the fire, and he began to ignore me, on top of showing how angry he could be on a daily basis. Not the best healing space to be in, but what could I do? I had quit my job. We couldn't sell the house in the incomplete condition it was in. I felt trapped. Anger had begun to be my constant companion, along with deep sadness and loneliness. My life felt empty, and I did not know how to make that emptiness go away.

Yet I persevered. The insightful walks in the forest always brought me to calm and peace and resolution for the time being. I listened to positive CDs and constantly worked on keeping good thoughts flowing, which was challenging when I walked into the house and looked around at the ugliness all around me. It was like trying to put my mind and imagination in a completely different place than the one I was really living in. How could I imagine feeling happy and healed when my life was so miserable? I didn't even know how to speak to my husband without making him angry, and my own anger was always simmering just below the surface, along with the tears, which were always able and willing to spill over.

One day we were arguing about how the house looked. I made my points about the constant unfinished renovations; his response was that it was *my* fault how the house looked! The audacity of his statement sent me into a state of uncontrollable rage I had never felt before in my life. I could feel my breath coming in great heaving gasps for air. A huge wave of energy began to work its way up my legs through the rest of my body. I began to shake violently in the grip of this incredible power. To my astonishment I saw my own two hands reach out and grab him by his sweatshirt and half pull, half drag him up eleven plywood steps, screaming at him the whole while. At the top of the steps I finally came to my senses and let him go. Stunned, I ran crying to the bathroom, where I sobbed for the better part of an hour. What was happening to me? How did I just drag my husband up all those steps?

I could not comprehend this bizarre behavior. Never before had I ever felt so unglued and so out of control—but at the same time I had never felt so free. It was scary to feel like I was losing my mind, but on the other hand, there was no turning back now, there was no escaping this radical energy that erupted out of my being. I could feel the rage coming through my body; it was always triggered by someone aggravating me or pushing me a little too far. It was always followed by an immediate feeling of freedom, of nothing being held back, of complete release.

Then came the numbness, the feeling that nothing mattered, of complete surrender, not caring about anything. Sometimes I sat and stared at the walls for hours, frozen in time, my arms too heavy for me to lift them to wipe the tears streaming down my face or the snot dripping from my nose, unable to hold on to any thought in this place of nothingness. It felt like I was being pulled into blackness, the big black hole of depression I had fought so hard to stay out of throughout my lifetime. Now it sucked me in and swallowed, digesting me into the deep bottomless pit like a fish being swallowed whole by a great white shark. My being felt captured by a big heavy net I could not get away from; the black waters held me under, and I drowned, having no strength and nothing to hold on to. This place of nothingness loomed around me: nothing to think, nothing to do, nothing to feel, nothing to be . . . just nothing.

After experiencing variations on this scenario over and over again, doubt reared its ugly head. Was I really healed? I tried to stay out of the great depression pit that had kept attempting to swallow me up ever since my teenage years. Many days I sat and did nothing while my mind raced with thoughts of all the things I *should* be doing. Some days I cried, but mostly I just sat feeling nothing; trying desperately to feel something . . . anything. I was so empty inside. Many friends called me almost daily throughout my breast cancer ordeal, but I felt utter loneliness. Then would come the rage. It would start to erupt through my body like a volcano, and I couldn't keep the lid on it anymore. I felt like I was losing my mind as this huge energy came up through me. My body would shake violently with each wave of emotion. I was completely out of control and out of answers. After these episodes, I would cry and feel lost and confused and ashamed.

After some weeks, the force of this rage seemed to lessen in intensity. I sat and stared into space, not saying or doing anything, my arms hanging limp at my sides. I didn't even answer the phone. I gave up the fight. I surrendered.

Then one day I woke up feeling really good. Nothing had changed, I just felt happy, for no reason, for the first time in my life. The feeling stayed. I started going for long walks and would imagine how I wanted my life to be and how I wanted to feel. I didn't know how or why this shift had happened, but I was ready to begin to *live* my life, not just exist in it. Nothing had changed in my outer world, the mess and plywood were still everywhere, only now there was peace in my being.

It was in this state of openness that I heard about a book called *The Journey*, by Brandon Bays. As I was listening to a teleseminar over the internet about cellular healing, the story came up of a woman—Brandon—who had, apparently, healed *herself* from a serious illness. The story immediately grabbed my attention, and I was compelled to read the book.

Her story, in so many ways, mirrored my own. She told of the huge energy that shook through her body and how it was through the opening and surrendering into these powerful emotions that she found release and healing. This resonated at my very core. My experience over the last year and a half had been a recognition of exactly that. Further, she went on to say that this emotional journey of healing was available to everyone, and could be undertaken in a matter of hours through guided processes that she had developed. I eagerly awaited my first Journey Intensive workshop and was not disappointed. It was to be the first step on my path to becoming a Journey Practitioner.

Through my Journey process work, I learned that my time of torment and grief had actually been part of my body's healing process, as the emotional toxins stored in my cells for a lifetime were at last released. I learned that the fears and doubts were scary because I had thought they, in some way, *were* the illness. Now I knew they were sim-

ply a natural part of me, free to come and go without hyp-
notizing or terrorizing me. I discovered how to open to
these emotions and to welcome them as a part of who I am,
and in that to find forgiveness and release. And in learning to embrace all my feelings, through my Journey processes I was finally able to break the deadly cycle of pushing
the rage down and then standing helplessly by while it
exploded. I was able to find peace.

The Journey is an integral part of the completion of my
healing. I no longer have doubt that I am completely healed,
and I find myself living life from a level of authenticity that I
could only have imagined before. To stay on my path, I meditate and spend time alone. I continue to allow the emotions
to flow through as they do and to stay focused on what I *do*
want in my life. I practice feeling the way I want to feel, and
I practice keeping my mind quiet when I don't want to feel
something. I also use all the tools I have learned about to keep
me on track in my life. Once a week I trade Journey sessions
with another practitioner. I want to keep myself as clear as
possible so I can keep living in each moment just as *I am*.

Through cancer I learned how to live in my body and
how to trust my body's wisdom. Through The Journey and
my natural healing process, I also learned how to love myself and how to live my authentic life. I am grateful every
day for the learning that continues to unfold and for knowing who I am—even if it did cost me a quarter of my beloved breast.

It is through The Journey that I have also discovered my
life's purpose: to share my story and Journeywork. I have

learned to love all parts of me—my slightly smaller breast, my scar, my anger, my fears—and I have been able to embrace the feeling of love I have for myself. It isn't selfish or arrogant to love oneself; it is *imperative*. It is my deepest prayer that we all find the freedom and healing available to each of us, and that we all live from this amazing place of awareness.

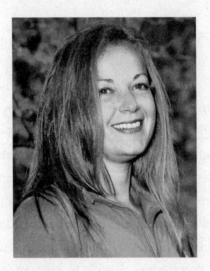

Susan D'Agostino *resides in British Columbia, Canada. She is an Accredited Journey Practitioner, Certified Conscious Coach, Health Coach and Emotional Freedom Technique (EFT) Practitioner. Susan specializes in working with cancer patients and those suffering from depression and anger issues. She teaches EFT at the integrated cancer clinic in Vancouver, BC. Her book* Hello Susan, It's Me, Cancer! *was written after healing from breast cancer using alternative and natural therapies and is available from her website at www.healingeverybody.com.*

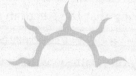

13

Who I Really Am

by Lesley Strutt

I originally began this chapter with a long dissertation on the quest for happiness: about how we all search for it and how it eludes us, and how I found it. And then my editing partner Pat Kendall called me to say what I already knew in my soul—that *that* was not what "my" chapter was about.

What I didn't want to share with you and everyone who reads this book—my children, my friends, my extended family members, my brother and sisters, cousins, aunts, uncles— is the raw story that carries the greatest exposure for me.

I created and perpetuated patterns of abuse in my life over and over until I finally saw the pattern and became determined to find out what was driving it. What was the root cause of choosing two husbands who mistreated me, the first physically, the second emotionally? What was at the core of my self-loathing? This is my story of addiction to creating situations in which I would and could play the victim. And it is the story of stopping the behavior, of turning and facing what I was running from. It is my journey to healing, to discovering that the freedom from such patterns comes from one place only—inside each of us.

I grew up in a noisy family with a mother who had a strong controlling personality and a father who mostly absented himself from us, either through work or just classically shutting us out. My mother raised us by the back of her hand. She loved us abundantly, too. I was the eldest, and I experienced my mother's depressions and illnesses during her pregnancies as something *I* should help mitigate. As early as age three, my mother told me, I would come to her and pat her knee, saying, "Don't worry, Mummy. Maybe tomorrow will be one of your good days."

My mother drank in the evenings. It was the age of alcohol and cigarettes. My parents gave huge parties, and the house would be filled with so much smoke you couldn't see from one side of the living room to the other. My mother's energy levels would dive after her drinking. The next morning, my father would head off to work, and she'd go back to bed.

She had a huge heart that wanted to love, but she was heavy-handed in her loving; loving, according to her way of being, included hitting when it was called for. She could reach back and smack you off your feet in the blink of an eye. My mother loved to tell the story of watching her dog, Wren, raise a litter of puppies and how, when the puppies got out of hand, Wren would bite them or growl, or put them in their place in another forceful way. So I guess you can say we were raised like puppies.

Fear of being out of control was the driving force in my mother's life; this translated into a desperate need to control every situation. Her anger about life and the things that were not going the way she wanted was a simmering rage that exploded often. As a very young child, I experienced ongoing terror for myself and for my siblings about this. It became a state of being, this terror. The other constant state was one of pure surrender to punishment. Any time she hit me, I would collapse into apologies—anything to stop the pain and receive a pardon for what I had done, real or imagined.

My mother and father had a volatile relationship. They were not a peaceful couple, so I vowed at an early age to find a husband to be peaceful with. By the age of sixteen I wanted to leave home; by eighteen, I was gone. I had a one-way ticket to Europe, some money and two girlfriends to travel with. We hitchhiked throughout the United Kingdom and northern Europe, wintered in Paris and went our separate ways in the spring of 1972.

By nineteen I was home, and quickly I looked for, and found, a way to leave again: I got married. That sounds cold, and I will agree. I remember having the thought, "I'll say yes to the first man who asks me to marry him." If I got married, rather than just living with him, I'd have the seeming safety of his commitment. The man I found was sweet in many ways, but he had a volatile temper that revealed itself very early on. I ignored it and continued to date him.

We met in our first year of university. His goal was to become a doctor and mine was to get my master's degree and teach. I was not friends with him. He was a good study partner, and we rarely needed to talk. The week before we were to get married, I was in the car with my dad on the way home from the university and I asked him, "What is love?" He said it was caring for the other person as much as you care for yourself. I puzzled over this answer and knew for a certainty that I didn't love the man I was marrying. "Oh well," I thought, "I'll give this a shot." Such a strange thought to have. Knowing I didn't love him, I had an instinctive sense that I was marrying him for an unclear reason and that the marriage wouldn't last.

My husband had a temper as vile as my mother's, so it was familiar. Our first physical fight occurred three weeks after we got married. We were washing dishes together, and I have no idea what I did or why the fight started. Suddenly he was shoving me backward toward the stairs—I thought he was going to push me down them. He stopped when I resisted, holding on to the top of the banister with all my might. I recovered and went for a long walk.

On that walk I had a conversation with myself. I remember thinking that I could leave him now and my life would be utterly different. But my mother had told me a few weeks before the wedding that if there was trouble in the marriage, I was not welcome to come home. I'd made my bed and now I'd make my life there. My littlest sister had moved into my bedroom, and there was no place for me anyway. My mother's words came back to me on that walk away from my husband. I stayed with him.

We *were* excellent study buddies—he became a successful medical doctor and I obtained my PhD, and in the midst of completing our degrees, we had two beautiful daughters. By the time our youngest daughter was two, he had one more year before completing his medical degree. We had very little money, so I rented one room in our house to a student. That also prevented my husband from hitting me and curbed somewhat his violent behaviors toward our girls.

He started dating other women. I was the bill payer, and I noticed on the credit card that there were dinners at restaurants that I didn't go to, and I asked him about it. And then he started telling me about parties he was going to and that I was not invited. When he attended a wedding in Toronto with his newest lover, I finally woke up.

The pain he was causing was so deep that I thought I might not survive. The day that it struck home I could barely function. I remember having to run an errand in the car; the girls were with me, and I have a vivid recollection of holding on to the steering wheel with all my might to keep the car on the road and not drive us headlong into oncoming traffic.

I recall watching a movie scene at that time where the young protagonist was standing in front of the sink in the bathroom, and he imagines cutting his wrists. I thought, "That's a dumb way to commit suicide. There are lots of easier ways." And I knew I could find them.

That thought woke me up completely. I accepted that I had two beautiful daughters to live for, and I chose to continue living. I went to the bedroom, woke my husband up and asked him to leave. And he did. The very next day! I was completely grateful.

I didn't blame my husband for our poor marriage; after all, I knew I had helped create it. And now I knew that love was the only way through the next part of my life. If I let love guide me, I would find my way. So I sent him blessings when he took a job in northern Ontario and his new lady love went with him. I sent her blessings, too. I sent myself blessings as much as I was consciously able to do . . . and finished my dissertation while working part-time and raising the little girls.

I met my second husband the following year, and we moved in together four years later. I look back now and see that this relationship was also not based on love; it was a relationship based on achievement on my part. He was very clear about what he wanted, and I did everything to meet his requirements. Mostly I considered what I did achieve to be a success—we raised four kids, traveled a lot, had a beautiful and unusual house, collected art and owned a luxury sailboat and many other trappings of a successful life.

I made what looked like a good marriage with him, but he never knew who I was. Not really. I crafted a life around being the wife he wanted and never contemplated the person I truly was. That marriage was full of loneliness and based on a different form of self-inflicted abuse: I allowed him to speak to me sarcastically and critically and laughed it all off. Our difficulties became unbearable when the girls reached their teenage years. As with my first husband, when he started to criticize the girls in an attacking, dismantling way, I stepped in, again and again. This caused him to complain that he was being ganged up on, and he would stop talking to me for days in order to punish me.

I came close to leaving him. We went to counseling, and though we never got to the root cause, it helped smooth things out. I stayed because it seemed that I was still achieving my goal of meeting his expectations and making a good marriage. Our marriage really ended when I gave myself permission to fail at this illusionary goal I had set for myself. In my deepest heart, I knew *I* had created this fictitious successful life, and it was up to *me* to step away.

My first step was a stumble, really. I betrayed my husband and fell in love with another man. The man, I later discovered, was married and had no intention of ever leaving his wife; but by that time I had left my husband and my life behind. Within the year, that man passed out of my life, and I had to live with the consequences of my actions.

This was the beginning of my journey into a dark abyss that had all the flavor of death. I was alone. I had broken the hearts of my husband and our large family. I had little access to my stepchildren and their children. I had left my marriage, my home and all my belongings. Who was I without those expressions of myself? They had been everything I lived for—an outward symbol of my happiness and success. I suffered a nervous breakdown and isolated myself from the world as much as possible. My life barely functioned.

And looking back now, I see how blessed I was. My boss gave me time off; my friends and two daughters and my sisters did their best to hold me in an embrace. As I slid into this abyss, I had a sense that I was not completely lost. Part of me was resting until I could take the first steps in healing. I was facing a truth that I had avoided my whole life—I didn't know who I was. I had loathed the person I seemed to be, and I had set up a pattern of building relationships with men who, in some way or other, treated me horribly. And I had let them. I gave them permission. It's as if I believed I was so worthless that I was being treated the way I *deserved* to be treated: "I *chose* this."

Now, for the first time in my life, I was really alone. I didn't know it, but the Universe was giving me the opportunity to find out what was at the heart of this pattern of self-abuse. What happened next brought me such clarity that I will never forget it for the rest of my life. And it was so simple.

My eldest daughter had been to an emotional healing seminar in Toronto and found it very helpful. She invited me to an event being given by the founder of the seminar series, Brandon Bays. The event was the launch of Brandon's book *Freedom Is*—and it was being held at a hotel ten minutes from my house in the Gatineau Hills, Quebec. Both the invitation from my daughter and the remarkable proximity of the location convinced me to go.

During the talk, Brandon asked us to turn to the person next to us and to say to them the words "You are a beautiful soul. I am honored to be in your presence. I love the person you are. You are an amazing soul." When my daughter looked into my eyes and said those words, my heart stopped. I saw the love in her eyes—but my whole body and mind rejected the words she was saying. I completely and entirely disbelieved her.

In that second, I knew that there was something deeply rooted in me that was preventing me from opening up and receiving her message of love. It was the first crack in the thick armor I had built around my heart.

I signed up for the upcoming Journey Intensive. Brandon's promise of freedom was compelling. I didn't know what it was freedom *from*, and I had no idea where this journey would take me. Nonetheless, I abandoned all caution. I packed my toothbrush and clean clothes (metaphorically) and set off on the greatest journey of my life—the quest for truth. The truth of *who* I really am.

The truth, when I found it, astounded me because it was so ordinary. And it just turned up. It turned up in a place I had been avoiding looking: right inside of my own self.

I began to go to more and more Journey events, peeling back layer after layer of behavior and story. Each time I got to another threshold, I wanted to pull back; I wanted to resist and push away the very thing that I knew was to be faced. And each time, I stood as still as I possibly could. And waited. Waited until my soul led me to the next layer of healing.

I was a person who, throughout my life, had shared so little of my private self that no one knew how I was really feeling. It was always masked under blanket statements such as "I'm fine." In the Journey workshops, we were invited to share in pairs what we were feeling and to step back into moments of the past that were haunting us. I did it. Again and again I took that terrifying path and experienced the exposure of the Journey process work. And again and again the reward was opening my eyes after the process and see-ing such compassion and love in the eyes of the person in front of me that true healing became a way of life for me.

Finally, in a Journey event in Ottawa, I was in a process with a young man who hit the nail on the head. I was doing a Physical Journey and found myself focused on the back of my knees. In fact, I experienced the sensation that my knees were being knocked at so my legs wouldn't hold me. My first images were of my ex-husband and how his sarcasm and criticism undermined me. But my Journey partner in-vited me to go back even earlier in time. And there sud-denly was a memory that shook me to my core.

I was about six years old, carving a pumpkin with my brother, who was three years old. My mom was evidently looking after my baby sister. We were out on the porch, and I was in control of the knife. My brother was very impatient. I had the thought in my head that if I could just finish the mouth he could do the eyes and the nose. But he didn't listen to my reasoning. He grabbed the knife from me and sliced his hand through the tendon between the thumb and forefinger. He screamed. I screamed. My mother came rushing and chaos broke loose. My brother had to go to the hospital. I was left at home to dwell on the terrible thing I had done even though I knew that it had not been strictly my fault. My experience of being the worst child in the universe was completely embedded in my body.

A terrible hatred of my mother was born in that long-ago moment. And a wall of such breadth had grown up between us that I had blocked any recollection of her speaking to me when she returned from the hospital. As I carried that ha-tred for her through my life, I cultivated a deep distrust of people. And I lived my life from a place where *I* was never to be trusted either. Nor would anyone ever love me again, because how could anyone ever love a girl who would cut her brother to the bone? That experience framed my whole life until I turned and faced my loneliness and self-loathing fully.

In the Journey process about my brother and my mother, I was able to completely forgive my mother for having caused me such pain. And I was able to forgive myself as well. In my mind's eye, I changed that toxic memory: now I saw my mother coming back from the hospital and hugging me, telling me that she realized that she shouldn't have given me such a big responsibility with the sharp knife. And I saw how I had blocked any of her words and gestures with my hatred and coldness.

Here at the very beginning of my Journeywork, I was offered a key to finding myself, and that key was *love*. The first Journey process Brandon teaches is to turn and embrace our emotions as they come and watch them as they melt away in the ocean of love that surrounds us at every moment. As I continued to process, I learned that everything that I was experiencing and that I had experienced was born in and came from *love*. And once I experienced and believed fully in the power of *love*, I had the first and most important treasure of my journey. It became my magic staff—I could point it at any dragon and say, "You are *love* showing up in dragon form. I am not afraid of you."

I signed up for the Journey Practitioner Program, and though I was not accepted into the program at first, that "no" gave me an opportunity to check my heart and find out what was really motivating me. Was it just to have more letters after my name, or was it for some deeper reason? I continued with the courses, knowing in my heart that I was on the right path for my quest. Eventually, in the face of financial challenges, the money showed up. With renewed confidence I applied again and was accepted immediately. I graduated from the Journey Practitioner Program, and that graduation meant more to me than any degree I had acquired in university.

The quest for happiness and freedom I had embarked upon led me to revisit many past memories that still triggered me, and to let go of my anger and misunderstandings. For instance, as I forgave my mom and saw truly that she was just doing the best she could at the time, all her loving I had blocked from my heart came flooding back. I saw that she truly did love me, and I opened my heart wide to recall and re-experience all the hugs and compliments I had rejected in the past. In forgiving my mother and many others whom I had shut myself off from, I found two more important keys to loving myself: forgiveness and gratitude. Forgiveness for being human, for doing the best that I could even if it was a lousy job, and gratefulness for the lessons that could be learned only because of the mistakes that had been made, mine and others'. What a healing that was!

I was now ready to look at my patterns of addiction and find out what had been motivating me to choose abusive relationships. I uncovered many negative and limiting beliefs about my worthiness and hidden vows I had made as a child, such as "I will never trust anyone again," that were running my life. I let them go. And each time I did, a part of me opened up, like petals on a flower. As my love of myself grew, so did my confidence. And this confidence in my own worth opened my heart to ask for and receive love in a wholesome manner, coming from a place of abundance instead of lack. And from this has come one of my greatest outer gifts: the amazing, loving relationship I have developed with my two daughters.

Kevin Billett offered his Visionary Leadership Program, and I signed up for that, too, determined to have a new way of experiencing relationships in my workplace. I am a research mentor for about one hundred active researchers in a university. I assist them in obtaining funds to finance their research projects, and the university counts on this money for its success as a research-intensive institution.

I headed off down that rocky, gnarly path of self-discovery again, and this time I encountered the monsters I created for myself in blaming others, playing the victim and defending myself. I met my outrageous control games and uncovered my compliance and rebellion patterns. I explored how they had served me and acknowledged what they had cost me.

With this freedom, I turned and faced how stress had been ruling my life at work. I opened into the possibility of what I would face if I failed completely and utterly at my job. How would that make me feel? In turning and facing that, I unhooked myself from an addiction to making myself indispensable to people at work. That double bind of being responsible for people's successes *and* failures was causing

me near nervous breakdowns every funding cycle. I chose
to stop it.

My first season at work following Visionary Leadership
II offered me an extraordinary opportunity to live in this
new way. My secretary fell ill and wasn't replaced until late
in the funding season. Then my father's health failed completely, and he was hospitalized. Without my secretary to
schedule appointments, I met researchers on a first-come-
first-served basis. My door was always open, and I reviewed
proposals in front of the researcher, in complete exposure
(without doing any of my normal homework and preparation), offered them comments and sent them on their way
to do the work. I visited my father in the hospital every
night, and I know that this time with him in his last days
was more valuable to me than any other time in our lives
together. He died eight days after my last proposal was
submitted—on deadline.

After working in this way in one season, I saw clearly
how I had previously created codependencies with my researchers. When the results from the season were in, we
had not done quite as well in terms of numbers of grants,
but we had secured more funds. The researchers who did
not succeed came to me with eager anticipation for the
next round. Instead of blaming me for their failure, they
said they had learned so much and were happy to resubmit.

My life continued to offer me surprises and extraordinary gifts. In the first half of 2010, I took a mini-sabbatical.
I found someone to look after my house, I found the funds
to cover my mortgage, and I took out a line of credit to pay

for a small apartment in Colorado where I had both friends and a love relationship that I wanted to explore more fully. I drove across the country with my little dog, my car packed with books, a few paintings, an air mattress, fold-up chairs, a couple of rugs and other treasures. My goal was to take time for myself and write the book that was tugging at my heart.

I arrived in Colorado on January 1. On January 5, I received an email from my lawyer saying that the neighboring national park was expropriating my house and I would have to sell. My world shook; the pain was acute. I realized I had two choices—get angry and fight this, or open into gratitude and hold myself in stillness while grace showed me what this was about.

As I held myself in deep stillness, it came to me how lonely I was in my house. It was on the edge of the park, far enough away from the city that my evenings were spent in solitude. I rarely came back into the city after arriving home. I also realized how tired I was of looking after an old house that took every penny of my savings to maintain. An historic building, it needed a huge amount of investment to be really looked after properly.

The house was the first example of a design innovation my architect father had pioneered in the 1950s, and I had been given clear indication that it could receive national heritage designation. I was in the midst of starting that process when I left for my sabbatical; my intention had been to start the process up again after my return. In opening to the possibility that grace was offering me a gift rather than punishing me, I saw that I could at least ask the national park to consider preserving the house. Architect friends contacted me to confirm this, and I wrote to the park accepting its offer and inviting representatives to consider the possibility of pursuing national heritage status for the house. They agreed. Let me say this: I know that this kind of creative thinking would not have been available to me if I had been playing my usual games.

The sale of the house to the national park raised a considerable amount of turmoil in my brother's life. He expressed a sense of injustice that I would potentially gain financially and sought the advice of a lawyer to force me to pay the family back for any help that the estate had given me through the years. This rift added to a deep wound in our family that had formed after my mother's and father's deaths.

To add to all of this, my love relationship ended. And though my lover's departure filled me with grief, I simply let it travel through my body with a deep sense of forgiveness and gratitude for what I had learned with him. And now, with all this happening, there was no other choice but to live from a place of complete surrender, where I was love, love was all there was, and everything that was taking place was taking place in love.

As time progressed, I realized that I needed to consider finding a place to live when I returned to Canada. I had a strong desire to have this settled before I returned to work in July, and I contacted a few girlfriends and asked their advice. One girlfriend wrote back to me in great urgency telling me that she had found me an apartment in a building near my work. She said she'd put my name on the list and informed me that I would love it, so to please call them and take it. I took the apartment, sight unseen. In July I moved into the apartment—and in August I met my true life's partner. We met walking our dogs near the apartment building, and the rest is history.

I have direct experience that whatever comes into our lives unexpectedly is truly a gift. The choice is ours whether we can open and receive it. Brandon shares this same message in her Journey Intensive when she describes opening into gratitude while facing the end of all she knew and held dear. I lived through something similar: I was invited to let go of everything and see what would turn up in its place.

I now know that there can be a great gift even in seeming disaster. And as I practice living from this new place of love, trust and vulnerability, every day I realize with renewed awe and wonder that *I am actually participating in my life.* Yes, there are challenges, and—yes!—love is here every day, especially in the face of those challenges. It's a strange land I live in now, where dragons turn into butterflies once I face them fully. I am not entirely comfortable in this new way of living, yet as I write these words, I realize that I don't care. Even when it is uncomfortable, I choose to live here in this new land of love and self-acceptance rather than to chase after mirages of false comfort in the desert of my old life.

When Pat told me that my chapter about the quest for happiness was not "my" chapter, she was quite correct. The truth is that happiness is a state just like any other. It moves, shapeshifts, transmutes. What truly centers me is the connection to who I really am, and that translates as an abiding sense of wholeness and well-being. Here is where I choose to live.

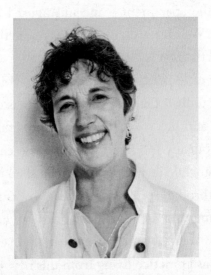

Lesley Strutt's *work with The Journey and Visionary Leadership grew out of her own experience of unhealthy stress and disempowerment at work. Her near nervous breakdown led her to realize that feeling powerless can lead to ill health and deep unhappiness, and her journey to wellness and confidence created a desire to share with others the tools she uses. As a Journey Practitioner and a Conscious Coach, her passion is to help people become conscious of the choices they make in life and access their true potential no matter what challenges they face. Contact Lesley at lesley@lesleystrutt.ca.*

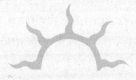

Afterword:
An Invitation from Brandon

I hope you have been as inspired and moved as I was in reading these healing stories. They genuinely are life transforming.

And now this is your invitation to begin your own healing journey.

Following this page will be a list of all the support and resources you will need not only to start your journey but also
to continue it. I have included The Journey's international and
North American office numbers so you can have that personal
contact, as well as our email and website details and an in-
troduction to what takes place in our various seminars—if
you feel called to really dive in. We give seminars all over the
world, and the chances are there may be one happening near
you, so please check out our website, where you will also find
a list of the Journey Practitioners who are available in your
area and who can help you experience the in-depth work.

I originally named this powerfully transformative work
The Journey because it *is* a journey, a lifelong journey. As you

can tell from the stories, it's not a onetime fix-up job, but an open invitation from your own heart to continue deepening in your realization of your own authentic self. It is deep work that clears the blocks, shutdowns and silent saboteurs that have held you back in life, and it is process work that puts the tools firmly in your hands so you can uncover your own truth and find your own answers.

This is the most liberating work I know of, and in reading these stories you can see it gets results! I always say, "The Journey can't give you anything. It's not a process of addition, but, rather, a process of subtraction. When you subtract the lies, the blocks, when you get to the root cause of what is running your show and clear it, when you clear the cell memories operating at an unconscious level, then the natural joy and love that is your own essence can shine."

In a nutshell, The Journey helps you to take the lampshade off your light, it allows you to awaken naturally to your deepest essence—to the love, the peace that is your own nature. It gives you the ability to wake up and heal your life, to live a guided life of authenticity and love.

So, following this page you'll find everything you need to get started—the Living The Journey Process designed specifically for this book, as well as some additional tips and wisdom from our authors along with their contact details.

It's time to open your heart, roll up your sleeves and begin your journey of a lifetime, and to uncover the love and joy that is your own essence.

Namaste,
Brandon

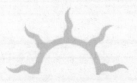

Important Contact Details

Worldwide website: www.thejourney.com

UK: International Head Office
The Journey, PO Box 2
Cowbridge, CF71 7WN
United Kingdom
Tel: +44 (0) 1656 890 400
Email: infoeurope@thejourney.com

The Journey North America Office
Email: info.na@thejourney.com
Tel: 1-855-625-6876 or 1-970-493-2111

Journey Outreach International
Email: info@journeyoutreach.com
Website: www.journeyoutreach.org

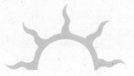

Seminars:
Information and Resources

The Journey Intensive
Real Tools—Real Healing—Real Freedom

Do you desire more fulfilling relationships with your loved ones, greater satisfaction in your career, improved health and well-being, spiritual growth?

The Journey Intensive with Brandon Bays is a two-day experiential workshop, giving you the tools to make the necessary life changes to move forward! Many participants describe this seminar as *"the most transformational experience"* of their lives. Drawing from direct, personal experience and sharing her inspirational story of healing and developing this life-transforming work, Brandon will guide you step-by-step through your own personal journey, teaching you The Journey Method that has transformed the lives of hundreds of thousands of people around the world.

During the Journey Intensive weekend, supported by a highly experienced team of Staff, Trainers and Practitioners, you will learn The Journey Method. Following a step-by-step

process, you will get to the root cause of long-standing issues
and get in touch with your own emotions, emotions you may
have shut down, numbed or denied for many years because of
past experiences or current circumstances such as stress, depression, relationship issues, work/life imbalance, illness . . .
allowing the possibility of physical and emotional healing.

You will use tools to:
- Access your true feelings.
- Learn how to deal healthily with your emotions.
- Uncover and clear the blocks and limitations that
  hold you back.
- Find completion and release years of baggage that
  has been weighing you down.
- Reconnect with your authentic self, your true potential.

You will experience:
- Inspirational teaching stories.
- Guided visualizations and meditations.
- Practical group work.
- One-to-one process work, with a partner of your
  own choosing.
- How easy it is to access your body's infinite wisdom.

In the course of the two days, you will also:
- Learn straightforward, repeatable tools to use in
  your daily life.
- Experience firsthand the benefits of clearing out
  stored issues.
- Let go of emotional baggage.

- Feel energized and inspired to continue living your life as your true potential.
- Find out how to access continued support through local grad meetings and ongoing programs.

To find out the dates of our Journey Intensives around the world, please visit us at **www.thejourney.com.**

The Journey Intensive is a deeply transformative event that gives you the freedom to live your life the way you always dreamed it would be. You've read these healing journeys. Now we hope you feel inspired to experience your own emotional and physical transformation and join us at our next event!

What people say about The Journey:

"I've evolved from Orphan Annie to *Annie Get Your Gun*. I feel like I'm a woman with a toolbox."

—*Annie*

"I am completely off all antidepressants, I feel like I have a life for the first time in over thirty years. This has worked for me where numerous other processes have completely failed."

—*Craig*

"A year on, my life has changed immeasurably. I've got the job I love, I'm married to a man I adore and have a much healthier lifestyle."

— *Janet*

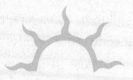

The Journey Accredited® Practitioner Program

Are you ready for the next step?
Then give yourself the gift of a lifetime!

Throw away the formulas and undergo deep process work. The Journey Accredited® Practitioner Program is a series of "hands-on" retreats that will teach you how to work and live energetically in consciousness, at the deepest level, with yourself, your loved ones or your clients. You will learn how to uncover your own deepest healing while becoming a competent facilitator in a professional setting.

There are seven courses, each designed to take you through The Journey Method™ to learn how to:

- Facilitate any journey for any person and any ego type.
- Combine neuro-linguistic programming tools with Journey processes to allow consciousness to clear out silent saboteurs.

- Manifest all of your heart's desires by clearing all of the soul's obstructions.
- Work with children, teenagers, the elderly . . . and work with anyone more fluidly.
- Uncover the real core issue underneath the surface story and get to the root of what blocks us.
- Work with a huge array of very specific issues, including sexual blocks, addictions, abuse, rape, illnesses, obsessions, relationship issues, depression, rage, shutdown and much more.
- Work more confidently with emotional resistance, in ourselves and with new clients.
- Live your life as a vibrant expression of grace, catalyzing healing on every level with everyone you touch.
- Uncover your soul's path for freedom in your Life's Purpose process, and help others uncover their own Life's Purpose.

The Journey Practitioner Program is the deepest program we offer and is perhaps one of the most in-depth programs for healing practitioners in the world. The best thing about becoming a Journey Practitioner is knowing how to live a guided life in conscious abundance. We look forward to welcoming you to this extraordinary healing work.

"How to put into writing healing stories using Journeywork; how to share about the marvelous, wonderful, unique tool that is The Journey? Where do I begin? How do I start to share what for me is a daily occurrence? Every day in my office I witness deep, lasting transformation. I see people freeing themselves from bouts of depression, allergies, anxiety, grief, low self-esteem, debilitating mood disorders and physical ailments, such as high blood pressure, IBS, migraines, even cancer!

"How do I describe the indescribable? Should I talk about the person who cleared herself of breast cancer in just two processes? Or the person who suffered from sexual impotence for as long as he could remember and was able to resume having a normal sex life again after just two sessions? Or should I talk about the one who was suffering from panic attacks and couldn't sleep but felt an instant relief and change after the first session? Or maybe I could talk about the lady who had been totally unable to let go of a past heartbreak to the point of becoming obsessive, and was able to forgive and move on? Or about the lady who had been unable to tend to her dying mother in the last days of her life, and was able to surmount her fears in one session . . . and was then able to let her go in peace while holding her hand? Or about those who were suffering from fibromyalgia to the point of being in constant pain and who are now pain free? Or do I talk about myself, finally released from the relentless, harsh, subtle, critical voice that kept me feeling 'never good enough' and unworthy, no matter what I did or how much I succeeded?

"As you can see, I am in awe of what I witness every day and am very, very humbled by it."

—Dr. Marie-Sylvie Roy, PhD, CPsych

"In my experience, when we essentially ask the Universe to 'use me,' the Universe says, 'Great—but first you need to undergo a life training!' For me the Practitioner Program was that life training. It completely changed my life 180 degrees. It gave me the confidence, the tools, the skills and the deeply liberating process work I needed to show up in life as my true self. It has allowed me to 'take my place in life,' to contribute to humanity, living from a place of forgiveness, love and compassion, not as a fanciful notion, but as a humbling, living, breathing life process. Nothing upon nothing has transformed my life and continues to do so like the Journey Practitioner Program."

—Laurie

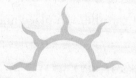

Stop the Food Fight

FOOD! Friend or Foe?

Have you ever:
- Tried a diet and it just didn't work?
- Joined a gym, paid the membership and after a few months simply stopped going?
- Looked in the mirror and criticized yourself for being too fat or too thin?
- Starved yourself in order to maintain that perfect weight?
- Obsessively counted calories only to gain more weight?
- Convinced yourself that you will start a healthy eating program tomorrow?

We all have a relationship with food, often unhealthy, and our eating habits are frequently driven unconsciously, beyond our control, by deep and perhaps long-forgotten emotional issues. These emotions, along with childhood memories and conditioned patterns, go unnoticed and sabotage any attempts we make to change unless we get to the root cause of what put them in place and clear them out.

It's Time to STOP the Food Fight!

This powerful three-day program with author and seminar speaker Kevin Billett will change your life by helping you:

- Get to the root cause of unhealthy eating behaviors.
- Clear out deep-seated emotional drivers.
- Uncover the major secret driver of your unhealthy consumption.
- Resolve issues of low self-esteem, poor self-image, lack of willpower and more.
- Stop the inner battle with food using practical, repeatable techniques.
- Create a healthy, liberating and lasting lifestyle.
- Make shifts to reach and maintain your goals.
- Come to peace, once and for all, with a supportive eating plan.

If you are ready for LASTING change, please visit www.stopthefoodfight.org or call our international or North American office. It could change your life!

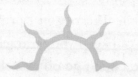

The Living The Journey
Process Overview

I am sure that if you are reading this, it is because you are feeling pulled to begin your own journey of healing and awakening. And to that end I have created a special clearing process, specifically designed for the readers of this book.

I have simplified and pared down the Emotional Journey process from the original book, *The Journey*, to its most essential elements, so that you can have a taste, a direct experience of this life-changing work. (If you are feeling pulled to experience the deeper, more comprehensive work, then get the book, *The Journey*, or better still, go to the website and find out about Journey Intensive workshops in your area, or call a Journey Practitioner living near you. With the support of Journey trainers and practitioners, you can undergo the more in-depth work at an Intensive or one-on-one.)

Before embarking on your journey, I recommend you set aside at least two hours of quiet time with a friend who can act as your partner in this. And before beginning, I suggest that you both read these detailed instructions at least twice so you can relax and just let the process flow naturally.

This is a process that *must* be done with another person or with a companion CD, so you can relax, close your eyes and turn within. The reason I prefer working with a live person is they can keep you on track and hold you to a high standard so you don't go off into the mind, but rather stay present to what is happening with your body, being and feelings. So it's best to work with a friend who has read this book and is willing to treat this as a divine experiment.

The process is predicated on you having already uncovered an emotion or pattern that you feel "hooked" by in some way—one that may be operating in the background or keeps arising, no matter how often you have tried to fix it or explain it away.

So when you sit down to do this process, be open with your partner and share with him or her what emotions have been coming up for you lately. Or if it is a pattern you recognize that you run, get still, soften your body and notice how that behavior makes you *feel* emotionally.

The process always starts with a feeling. Once you've opened and allowed the feeling to arise, to be fully felt, you will feel yourself opening down through various emotional layers and will finally end up in what I call "Source"—the boundless infinite presence of love, peace, joy, freedom, everything. This that is the core of your being, that is your own soul (and you know you are resting in Source when it is omnipresent, everywhere).

While resting in Source, you will then be asked to go two layers deeper by "opening into the very heart of it and expanding."

Then you will go to a "campfire," and at this campfire you will welcome a younger you of any age or age range. You will also invite the present-day you, as well as a mentor whose wisdom you trust and any people who have contributed to your having felt the emotional pain you started with. At the campfire, you will have a chance to dialogue out loud together, letting the younger you finally get a chance to empty out all the unspoken words, stored emotions, unvoiced pain, hurt, shame, blame, etc., and then those with you at the campfire will be given the opportunity to respond. This dialogue of "emptying out" will finish when both the younger you and the other person feel completely emptied out, having fully voiced what's been there. Then the same opportunity will be given to the present-day you, and once again you will have the chance to fully empty out what had never before been spoken or expressed. Again, the other person will respond.

Then, when everyone is completely empty, has completely dialogued and spoken all that needs to be said, there is the invitation to forgive. The younger you forgives the other person, the present-day you forgives them, and then the other person forgives you, and finally you forgive yourself. So forgiveness happens all around to everyone at the campfire.

The campfire disappears, and you are once again resting in the vast boundless presence of love and stillness that is your own essence (Source). Next you will be guided into a "future integration" where your partner will check with your body that over time the healing will continue.

So you will hear your partner inviting you to "Step into the future a day from now and feel how you are feeling, breathe how you are breathing and open into the consciousness of you a day from now." And you will be checking in with your body a day, a week, one month, six months, one year and finally five years into the future—checking at every step of the way that the body and the being indicates it is willing to integrate and heal these old issues.

Then when you are five years down the line, staying open in that free consciousness of the future you, you will be asked to write a letter to the present-day you to give yourself some practical advice on how to live your life from the freedom, forgiveness and wisdom that is here. You will then open your eyes and let your own wisdom pour itself onto a page.

So in a nutshell the process looks like this diagrammatically speaking:

Emotion

Down
through
emotional
layers

Rest in Source
Campfire
Future Integration
Letter to Self

Let's go over it again in greater detail.

It is good to start by taking a few deep breaths in, consciously softening the body so you can *feel* what's coming up for you emotionally. Our emotions reside in our bodies, not our heads! So, during the process it is important to be present to what is happening emotionally *in* your body.

After softening the body you will simply welcome the emotion that you are feeling to fully arise, welcoming it to come up through the body. You will notice where it seems to reside most strongly, and then your partner will ask you to "Just surround this feeling with your own love, your own acceptance and softly open into the very core of the emotion and stay there." Then your partner will ask you, "What's in the core of this feeling? What's deeper? . . . What's coming up?" And the next layer of emotion will arise naturally.

Some of our feelings are very subtle, some strong, so it is important to just be open and present with your body to feel what is coming up.

At some point you may get to a layer devoid of emotion—where there seems to be a vast emptiness or nothingness or a haze or fog. I call this layer "the Unknown Zone," and it shows up differently for different people. Sometimes it can show up as a void or numbness or stuck-ness. Not to worry, this is a very natural layer for all of us to experience. If you find yourself in a field of nothingness, just know it is another layer and that beneath it lies the light, the love, the peace that is your essence.

If it does show up (and it doesn't always do so) then you will hear your partner give special instructions for someone who is in the Unknown Zone—words that will cause you to relax, open and "drop" through into your essence, into Source. If a "lid" shows up you will be asked to "peel" the lid back, and again you will feel yourself opening quite naturally and easily into your own self. If numbness or stuckness shows up you will be reminded that this is just another emotional level, and you will be asked to simply welcome it all and keep opening deeper.

The wording for all this (should it occur) is in the script, which I trust you will familiarize yourself with completely (by reading it several times) before actually undergoing the process.

Eventually you'll keep going down through all emotional layers (there is *not* a set number—it could be two layers or it could be eight or more!) into Source, into the boundless, infinite presence of oneness at the core of your being.

Then you will be invited to go to the campfire, and the nature of the campfire is unconditional love, peace. It's a forum where you can feel safe in finally emptying out what it is that you never spoke out loud before, or never even knew was stored inside. It is important that the entire process be done **out loud** (you've heard the expression "better out than in"), and what takes place is a dialogue where everyone at the campfire gets a chance to fully empty out what they never voiced before. When the dialogue occurs, I am always amazed at what comes out of my mouth. I never knew all those words, all those emotions, all those feelings, all that pain was stored there inside. I give the younger me the opportunity to really open up and let it all out!

It is important that you let the younger you speak in the voice of the younger you, because the truth is, the older you—the present-day you—has all kinds of wisdom that the younger you didn't have at the time, so it is very important for the younger you to *fully and openly* express what was **not** said at that time. The campfire is a time of honest, naked, raw exposure—letting the younger and present-day you speak the open truth about how you felt at the time.

Then the other person has a chance to speak, and the dialogue continues until both parties are fully empty.

Then the same dialogue takes place for the present-day you, and both people empty out completely, when you will be invited to forgive. First the younger you forgives, then the present-day you, then the other person forgives and ultimately you forgive yourself. It's a forgiveness fest.

It's important that the forgiveness is real, heartfelt and complete. If you find you can't forgive, then it is probably a signal you are still holding on to something—some unspoken words or some feeling you weren't willing to admit to yourself. So when working with your partner, please encourage each other to be totally real and to *fully* empty out at the campfire.

Of course, there is a mentor present, so when in doubt, ask the mentor, "What would have to happen in order to forgive fully?" Then let that take place so the forgiveness can be completely true and heartfelt. When all is fully forgiven and you've received any final advice from your mentor, then the campfire disappears and everyone merges into the light.

Next you will be taken into the future integration, by stepping into the future and checking with your body and being at every stage. You will notice that as time goes on you are feeling more whole, more complete, lighter, freer.

And finally, at five years down the line, you will be asked to write a letter to yourself, and your partner will hand you a blank sheet of paper. You will open your eyes when all parts of you are fully integrated and then just let your own wisdom fall effortlessly onto a page.

This whole process will likely take about forty-five minutes to one hour, and following it you might like to thank your partner, get a cup of tea and then switch, so they too have a chance to undergo this divine experiment.

The key here is to trust yourself, trust the process, trust life. Know that your body, your being *wants* you to come home, it wants you to heal. So just be innocent like a child and let it all unfold naturally and easily.

With this process (unlike the Emotional Journey from the original Journey book) there is nothing for your partner to write down. Instead, they will simply read the process with you, be present to you, feel with you, down through the emotional layers, through the Unknown Zone (if it occurs) into Source.

Then they will accompany you through the campfire, encouraging you to be open, honest, to *really* empty out all of what's stored in your body, your heart, your being. And then they will encourage you to forgive.

The campfire disappears and, innocently, by stepping into the future, you will keep checking with your body and your being that over time the healing will occur. And finally you will write that letter from the future you to yourself.

It's a powerful, deeply transformative process, especially when you decide to be open, real and honest. So just decide to give it a shot. You have nothing to lose but some old baggage . . . and everything to gain from taking that old lampshade off your light.

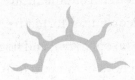

The Living The Journey
Process Instructions

Before starting the process, share with your partner what has been coming up for you lately—what emotions and patterns you have noticed. Once you've identified and are *feeling* a fairly strong emotion, you can begin the process. You can close your eyes, take a few deep breaths in and let your awareness come to your body (where all emotions are stored). Take a few moments to soften your body, let any resistances fall away and open your heart, your being. Be fully present with yourself, with your emotions, with your body.

Your partner, the processor, will read to you the two "down through the layers" paragraphs, repeating them at every emotional layer until you open into Source or the "Unknown Zone." They will know you are in Source when it is inside, outside, everywhere—omnipresent; and then they will take you two layers deeper by going into the heart of it and expanding.

If you come across a layer of emptiness, blackness, blank, fog, haze, etc., then they will read the Unknown Zone instructions to you. Or if you find a lid or feel stuck or numb, they will read the directions about peeling the lid off, and you will find yourself beginning to open in Source, where you will be taken two layers deeper.

This will be followed by the campfire, the future integration and a letter to yourself.

Have the intention that you will be open, innocent, exposed and trusting. You can even begin by breathing into those qualities.

So take this moment to be very real, take down any armor or defensiveness and be willing to be nakedly exposed. Just open right now and allow all the feeling that is here to arise, and you can both start.

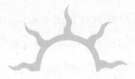

The Journey Process

Down Through the Layers

Processor: (Read the two "down through the layers into Source" paragraphs below to your partner over and again until they are resting in Source. If they uncover an Unknown Zone or lid, read those instructions and they will take your partner into Source. So begin by asking:)

"What feeling is arising?" *(Let them name the emotion . . . then say:)* "Just allow all of the feeling to come flooding . . . it can be allowed to come even more fully . . . Now surround the feeling with your own love, your own acceptance and then feel yourself opening, going right into the very core of it as you ask yourself, What's in the core of it? . . . the very center of it? Or, What's beneath it? . . . and just stay there . . . So what's here? . . . What's even deeper than this or what's rising up into this?" . . . *(Let them name the new feeling, remember to give time . . . once they name the new feeling, say "Great" and continue.)*

"Now just allow all of this feeling to come flooding . . .

Really welcome it. As it becomes fuller ask, What's in the core of it or what's beneath it? . . . and then surround it with your own love, your own acceptance and feel yourself opening right into the very center of it . . . and just stay there . . . So what's here? What's rising up into it? . . . What's deeper?" . . . *(Let them name the next feeling; say "Great," and then continue repeating these two paragraphs down through the layers until they open into Source.)*

Unknown Zone Instructions

Processor: (If they arrive in nothingness, blackness, emptiness, a haze or fog, read the following:) "Great! You are in the Unknown Zone, and you know what your job is—just to relax and welcome it. It's just another layer . . . So tell me, what's it like?" *(Let them describe it and be encouraging.)* "Are there any edges or boundaries anywhere, or does it just go on and on?" . . . *(Encourage them to check it out and describe it and then ask:)* "What's coming into this vast field of nothingness, this emptiness? . . . What's seeping in now? . . . What's coming through the cracks, the pinholes? . . . What's beginning to suffuse this blackness?" *(Let them speak out loud—usually it's light, love, peace, calm, some Source-like word. Then say:)* "Just feel yourself opening and expanding right into the very heart of it . . . So what's here?" . . . *(Give time for them to identify what's here, then say:)* "Great! So as you feel yourself expanding just ask yourself, What's in the heart of this?" . . . *(Let them answer and then say:)* "Just feel yourself opening and expanding in this" . . .

(Keep repeating the above paragraph until they are resting in Source, which is a presence that is everywhere.)

Lid or Stuckness Instructions

Processor: (If there is a lid just have them peel the lid back and ask:) "What might it be covering or protecting you from feeling? . . . What's beneath it? . . . Just feel yourself opening into it . . ."

(Then continue with the Unknown Zone instructions until they open into Source.)

Source

Processor: (Once they arrive in Source, in a presence that is omnipresent—inside, outside, everywhere—then take them two layers deeper by repeating the paragraph below.)

"What's in the heart of this, the very core of this? . . . Just feel yourself opening and expanding into this."

(Then say:)

"Just rest in this infinite vast expanse that is your own essence."

Campfire

(Processor says:) "Now imagine a campfire, the nature of which is unconditional love and acceptance. To this fire, welcome a younger you—it can be any age range from zero right up to now. Then welcome to this fire the present-day you. Also at this fire is a mentor whose wisdom you trust. It can be a saint, a sage, an enlightened master—someone in whose divine presence you feel safe and whose wisdom you trust.

"Now welcome to the fire specific people who may have somehow played a part in all the painful emotions you first started this process with. You can invite as many as you like, but for the sake of today's process, you will likely only get a chance to speak with one of these people."

"So who's here?" *(Let them answer.)* . . . "Does anyone else need to be here?" . . . *(Let them answer.)*

Dialogue and Empty Out

(Processor says:) "Sitting with your mentor in the presence of this protective fire of unconditional love, I'd like to speak to the younger you. This younger you has gone through a lot of painful emotions *(you can even name them)*, and it's time to give the younger you a voice: a chance to really empty out all of these strong feelings that you may previously not have felt safe to express, feelings that you may not have had a chance to speak out before, and let the other people at the campfire open and listen. Let the younger you or the mentor choose which person sitting at the fire you wish to speak to.

"So if the younger you could speak from the heart, really open up and let come up and out what needs to be said, to get it all off their chest and out of their cells, what might the younger you say? . . . Let the younger you empty it all out." *(Make sure they speak out loud. Give plenty of time to answer, be encouraging and ask them to speak in the voice of the younger them, in the first person, and once emptied, then say:)*

"Knowing that the other person was probably doing the best they could with the emotional resources they had at that time, what might they respond if you could give them a voice? . . . Let them speak *not* from the ego or personality, but from some deeper place . . ." *(Be encouraging. Let them respond.)*

"If the younger you could respond, what might you say?" *(Let them empty out.)*

"And if the other person could respond, what might they say?" *(Again, let them respond.)*

*(Keep dialoguing and continuing to empty out until both parties are **completely** empty.)*

"Now ask if the mentor has anything that needs to be said. What might the mentor say?" *(Let them answer.)*

"Now it's time to go to the present-day you . . . And if the present-day you could really open up, get it all off your chest, out of your cells, what might the present-day you say to this other person?" *(Let them answer.)*

"And if they could respond, what might they say?" *(Let them answer.)*

(Keep dialoguing until all are empty . . . then ask:)

"If the mentor had anything to offer, what might the mentor say?" *(Let them answer, then say:)*

"Is there anything else that needs to be said by anyone in order to feel complete? If so, let them speak that now." *(Let them empty out more if needed.)*

Forgiveness

(Processor says:) "Now asking the younger you, even though you might not be able to condone the other person's behavior, even if it's totally unacceptable by *anyone's* standards, I'd like to ask you if you'd be willing to forgive the *soul* of the other person from the bottom of your heart." *(Let them answer.)* "Then go ahead and forgive them in your own words, out loud, from your whole heart." *(Let them forgive.)*

"And then ask the present-day you the same: even if you in no way condone this other person's behavior, even if it's not acceptable by *anyone's* standards, are you willing to completely and utterly forgive the soul of this person with all your heart?" *(Let them answer.)* "Then go ahead and forgive them in your own words, wholeheartedly, out loud." *(Let them forgive.)*

"Now if *you* need to be forgiven for any reason, let the younger you open your chest and let the other person forgive you wholeheartedly . . . And you can let the present-day you do the same.

"Now it is time to let that person and any others sitting by the fire merge into the light, with a prayer for them that somehow they can find forgiveness for themselves . . . So go ahead and send them that prayer as they merge into the light." *(Let your partner speak aloud this prayer in their own way.)*

"And now there is just the younger you, the present-day you and the mentor here at the campfire, and there is still a short dialogue that needs to take place here.

"So letting the present-day you turn to the younger you and repeat after me: I am so sorry for all the previous pain you went through . . . You just didn't have access to the wisdom that I do now . . . and I promise you will **never** have to go through that previous pain again . . . because from now on I will love you and protect you . . . and you can have access to this wisdom, this love, this forgiveness any time you like . . . and I forgive you for anything you need to be forgiven for.

"Now hugging the younger you, let the younger you merge inside, growing up now in this love, acceptance and forgiveness.

"And turning to the mentor and asking the mentor if there is any final communication the mentor might like to make before merging into the light." *(Let them answer.)* "Then let the present-day you and the mentor merge and dissolve into the boundless presence of love that is your own essence, your own soul—this infinite field of Source. And just allowing your own awareness to expand and become spacious, vast, open and free in front of you . . . letting it become boundless, free and endless behind . . . spacious to all sides of you . . . and just resting now in the boundless presence that is your own essence."

Future Integration and Letter to Self

(Processor says:) "Staying wide open in this boundless presence of love, of light that is your own essence, I'd like to ask you to step into the future a day from now . . . Breathe how you are breathing, feel how you are feeling and open into the consciousness of what you are feeling right now . . . It's you a day from now . . . How are you feeling? . . . Check your body . . . Is that old issue here anymore?" *(Let them answer.)* "Great!

"Now step into the future a week from now. Breathe how you are breathing, feel how you are feeling, open into the consciousness of you a week from now. How are you feeling? . . . About yourself, about life?" . . . *(Let them answer.)* "Great!

"So now step into the future a month from now. Breathe how you are breathing, feel how you are feeling, open into the consciousness of you a month from now. How are you feeling? . . . About yourself, about life?" . . . *(Let them answer.)* "Check your body . . . Is that old issue coming up any more or is it disappearing altogether?" *(Let them answer.)*

"So now step into the future six months from now. Breathe how you are breathing, feel how you are feeling, open into the consciousness of you six months from now. How are you feeling?" . . . *(Let them answer.)* "Six months down the line over 70 percent of your cells have already healed, so how *are* you feeling? . . . About yourself, about life?" . . . *(Let them answer.)* "Check your body. Is that issue arising or is it completely gone?" . . . *(Let them answer.)* "Great!

"So now stepping into the future a full year from now. A year from now there will not be a single molecule in your body that was here today—you are *literally* all new. So breathe how you are breathing, feel how you are feeling, open into the consciousness of you a year from now. How are you feeling? . . . About yourself, about life?" . . . *(Let them answer.)* "Check your body. Is that old issue even coming up anymore, or is it completely gone?" . . . *(Let them answer.)* "Great!

"And now step into the future five years down the line. Breathe how you are breathing, feel how you are feeling, open into the consciousness of you five years from now. How are you feeling? . . . About yourself, about life?" *(Let them answer, be encouraging.)*

"Now staying wide open in this consciousness of the future you, I'd like to ask the future you if you might be willing to write a letter to the present-day you, giving yourself practical advice on how to be, what to do, how to live *from* this consciousness. It is said the fact that you can even conceive of this consciousness means you can start from here, starting now. So you'll find you'll be able to open your eyes *only* as soon as all parts of you are fully integrated, and when all parts of you *are* fully integrated and willing to carry on the healing process naturally on its own, you *will* be able to open your eyes and let your own wisdom pour itself onto a page, letting the free, wise future you guide you now. So you can open your eyes now when you are ready and let this letter to yourself fall onto a page."

(When they open their eyes, hand them a blank sheet of paper and a pen so they can write their own letter to themselves. Make sure you thank them, praise them and share what a gift it was to work together in this way. Then if you'd like, you can switch.)

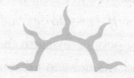

Tips from the Authors

Life goes on. And how do we who have written this book, as Journey Practitioners and Conscious Coaches, stay in the flow of life, of grace, of love, of peace—of Source—when the waves of this world buffet us, and there is not a Journey class or process to be had? What do we do to stay clear and on purpose, to find the courage to move forward when life is not going as we would have it go?

Here, alphabetically by author's first name, are the activities, awarenesses and processes that we use day to day, to stay on track and enjoy our lives as the works-in-progress that we are. Some of them will seem familiar, as they were included in the authors' chapters; others are new. We hope some of these tools will be helpful for you, too, when the waves get big—or even when they don't. Enjoy!

Arsene Tootoosis:
I know in my heart and in my actual experience that our ceremonies and Journeywork fully complement each other. I continue to live fully and embrace this way of life

and the tools I have that help me. *I attend the Inten-sives* that we have secured in Saskatoon every six months. *I continue with my self-care daily*. And I *work with oth-ers.* It is great to see people dive into the process work and find forgiveness and freedom in whatever issues are pre-sent for them.

Bet Diening-Weatherston:
I show up in life, I use any and all the tools I can get my awareness connected to, for myself and for others. I run through the trails, I crank up the tunes and dance like nobody's watching. I say outrageous things to make myself and others laugh . . . laughing is so good for the soul, I believe it heals all. I make dates with my husband, my son Jorin and my son Connor and I celebrate . . . *I live in grat-itude* even when I'm in a pissy mood because that too is welcome.

The tool that I use to stay clear and focused on a regular basis is to *challenge my "Can't List."* I keep an ongoing list of things that I feel I could not ask help for, figure out who I couldn't possibly ask that help from, and then go ask them for that help. WOW! . . . What a difference that has made in my life. The mere fact that I recognized my game of not asking for help brought to light a network of belief systems that weren't even consciously adopted as my own. So when I hear myself saying "I can't, or shouldn't or no way . . . ," I stop and wonder, "Is this really true? What would it take for me to actually bust through the limiting beliefs that hold me back in life?"

Cynde Sawyer:

How do I help myself stay in this understanding? First, to help me really live this, *I keep in touch with those who support the understanding that story does not define any of us.* This actually helps. Also in a meditation, my father's spirit came to me and "said," "We have danced this dance before. Sometimes I lead and sometimes you do. Just like a single dance in your lifetime is insignificant, so is this lifetime. It is like a gnat in the universe." I really get this. So *I remind myself that the story of this lifetime is so insignificant that one event or relationship is not worth getting upset over.*

I put out a prayer to be with like-minded people, and my prayer has been answered with many Journey people, both practitioners and clients, who are like-minded. Interesting also is that those who seemed not likely to understand how I have evolved and who I have become, really do understand. Yes, there are people in my life who look like they would like to hang garlic around me or tell me this is all bull. I love them and smile and let it go. I do not have to prove anything, I am free.

And finally, what keeps me centered is *gratitude.* I never really understood the power of gratitude before I started this work. Sure, I was glad when my son was doing okay, and that my other kids were okay, etc. However, the deep feeling of gratitude that I now experience surpasses anything that I felt before. My heart swells with the feeling, it is so enormous; *I am grateful for large things and also for the small things in my life.*

Debbie Clarke:

The first tool I call my *"bullies" technique*. One morning when I awoke I was lying in bed thinking about a difficult situation that I was facing, not having a clue how to deal with it. I became aware of the very negative self-talk that I was hearing in my mind. I am á very visual person; when I closed my eyes I could see that the answers that I needed were in a vault. Standing in front of the vault was a gang of bullies—and they were all aspects of me. There was the bitch, the self-doubter, the pessimist and many other self-defeating and negative aspects of myself. They were being very verbally abusive to me. So I imagined in my mind's eye going up to each one of them, and with all acceptance and love, I asked them, "What is it you need?"

As with all bullies, they were acting tough to cover fear and insecurities, when they were actually seeking love and acceptance. When I gave them each the acknowledgment and love that they desired, they each softened and said they were sorry and that they were just trying to protect me. They stepped aside and I was able to open the vault with all the answers inside. The biggest answer was, "Just love and accept every aspect of yourself, and you can do anything that your heart desires." I realized that the parts of me that I had originally thought to be a weakness or a drawback, can be assets and strengths. Stubbornness can become determination, obsessiveness can be an eye for detail, skepticism can be the voice of reason and so on. When we love and accept all parts of ourselves, we can blossom into the greatness that is our true essence.

Another technique that I use for myself is that when I find myself struggling or feeling mentally or physically uncomfortable, *I take a moment to get still and ask, "What's here? What are you **really** feeling?"* When I name it and give it attention, it loses its grip on me and loses its power. It's like the boogeyman in the closet: once exposed, he isn't scary anymore.

Ilene Beal:

Aside from receiving Journey processes, I stay in this open energy primarily by using **mini-meditations**. I have learned I can get centered and grounded by taking a deep breath in, and exhaling out . . . then another . . . then turning my attention inside and just getting still. I can do that driving down a freeway, at my kids' ballgames, in any stressful situation. Then I get connected.

If there's still residue from an event or a crisis or just the world's noise and bustle, *I ask myself, what needs to happen here?* Is there something I need to do? Something I need to say? And then I follow my own answers, heard in the stillness.

Jared Beal:

How do I stay in this peaceful place? I turn off the radio and relax and reconnect with who I am in a *daily meditation*: *I just let everything go, get into that place of Being and rest there for a little while.* And the biggest thing I do is to *keep going back to Journey events and sharing my story with others*, letting that trigger things I still need to clear, and triggering things for the others, too. I love to share my story now. Yes, I'm grateful The Journey helped me to heal my back without surgery and keep the job that I love to do. And I'm even more grateful for all the healing I didn't expect: the gift of my wife, my kids and my whole self.

Jasmine Iwaszkiewicz:

There are times when I feel that I have somehow fallen off the "love wagon," and when this happens my body makes it crystal clear to me. I have learned to listen to this instrument, this navigation tool, this body—I have come to know fully that this body will always lead me into love, clarity and peace. When I am in my mind or out of a state of love—for the mind does not "feel" and as a result cannot fathom or feel love—*I breathe. I become very still, and I do what I call "opening into my body."*

I place one of my hands on my heart and I breathe into this tender and open heart space. I pay attention to it by placing all of my awareness in it. I listen to it, and if it tells me that sadness, fear or anger is here, I allow it to express itself through this body. If tears come, I welcome them all until nothing remains but stillness, peace and love. This feeling is vast and expansive, and my body becomes open once again, and my heart and mind indicate this to me through their calmness and peace.

I consider my thoughts, for I know that if I am in a state of worry or anxiety, it was born of some thought-process that led me down misery lane . . . and that my body has responded accordingly and lovingly by some signal. Whether that signal be an ache, a stomach pang, a headache or a sore back, the body talks to me in a myriad of ways and I have learned to interpret its signals by paying attention—just as one might do with a newborn baby. We learn that their differing sounds and cries mean differing things; that this newborn child has a need it wants to communicate so that we can offer our comfort, nurturing and support.

I also listen to music that makes me feel good. Sometimes this music has me dancing in my home or car. At other times it is soft and gentle and speaks of love and consciousness.

I no longer watch the news or read the dailies. I am unwilling to program my body or mind with fear, anger or war. I regularly recommend this one particular tool to my clients, and some of them ask me, "What do you talk about, then?" I tell them that I speak from my heart about what matters most—life, love, freedom and joy.

I have fun. I dance, play, sing, laugh, and am very much like a child in many ways. *I am always keenly aware of the beauty that is all around me,* and *I honor and respect myself.* It is from this place of self-regard and knowing that I interact with others and the world as a whole.

Lesley Strutt:

These are the tools I use daily:

Daily meditation: I begin in bed when I wake and say, "Thank you." This brings me into relationship with my breath, with my life force. I thank my body as I get up; my feet, my ankles, my legs and hips, etc. I bring myself into connection with my heart, scanning my body for any glitches or sticky parts and if I find any, I thank those parts and promise them I will listen. I will find time in my day to hear what they are saying to me. This is particularly helpful if I am going to work. I am then brought into harmony with my sticky parts and they don't keep showing up for attention throughout the day. They know I will find time to listen before ending the day.

Mantra: In the face of every challenge I access my heart song—*I love you. I am sorry for bringing you into this energy exchange, and I take full responsibility for my creative powers. Please forgive me* (especially if someone else was negatively involved in my newest creation). *Thank you, thank you, thank you.* This mantra is my version of the Hawaiian practice of Ho'oponopono, and I find it deeply healing for me and for the others involved in my created challenge.

Practice: I give and receive Journey processes regularly. I meet with friends who are conscious and share what is coming up in my life as I open to what is coming up in theirs. I honor everyone I meet because I know that everyone and everything coming into my life is created for my highest and best good from *love*, for *love*.

Insight I hold in my heart: I see myself like a plant. I grow, I flower and my petals fall to the ground. I turn brown and deteriorate, and all attachment to whatever I was that day dies away. Into that fertile ground all possibility (Life) can send its roots. So each day for me now is like a new beginning and a new death, or ending. And that is how I live my life, always curious to discover what new life and possibilities will be born every day.

Emotions: I treasure each emotion I experience and consider it a door-knocker to my soul. When an emotion comes
up, I welcome it, I observe it, I embrace it. If the moment is
a good one, I will open up the door and step through. If the
moment is less than ideal (for instance, if I am in a meeting),
I pause and feel the emotion, give it silent, brief attention
with the promise to sit with it later that day, say at bedtime.
I know it is here for me, to show me something.

Forgiveness: I offer myself forgiveness every day as my
love offering to myself and God. Internally I give forgiveness to, and ask for forgiveness from, everyone I have had
contact with during my day.

Patricia Kendall:

Here are four things that help me:

The first is a mantra: "If it's here, it's perfect." As a
former seeker of perfection, I have had to learn that perfection is not "someday, somehow, somewhere." It is now.
And now. And now. And now. The entire Universe, I have
learned through experience, is conspiring to bring me (and
everyone else) exactly what will most serve us in this moment. The packaging—good-appearing or bad-appearing
events, sad or joyful news, supportive or obstructive people, irritating or uplifting encounters—all that packaging is
irrelevant. As I look for the particular gift-with-my-name-
on-it that is sitting in each event-package, I move from reaction into gratitude, even before I have seen the gift, and
this serves me. And bringing this mantra into consciousness
helps me focus on the gift-to-come even before it shines
through its disguise.

The second is a practice from another discipline: the art of moving into vibrational peace with another through Ho'oponopono, or internally asking for forgiveness. When someone is irritating or hurting me, I have drawn that hurt or irritation into my life, so in some way I am participating in the anger or attack I feel I am receiving from the other person. And when I am irritating someone else, I have also drawn that circumstance to me. How to uncover the gift? When I feel on the outs with someone, whenever I remember, I internally repeat the Ho'oponopono prayer: "I love you. I am sorry. Please forgive me. Thank you." And something eases. In me? In the other? Does it really matter? I find peace, and usually I am not the only one. In this space-between-us-which-is-consciousness, I am One with the other. We both heal.

The third is an exercise in letting go of my two biggest peace destroyers: fear and anger. When my mind goes story-spinning into the past of blame or the future of worry, avoiding the feeling that is here now, here's what helps me bring it back and calm it down:

1. *I catch the mental "story."* This type of inner story tends to feel charged with anxiety, worry, fear, regret, guilt, anger, etc. I listen for phrases like "If only I . . ." "What if . . ." "How could he/she/you/they . . ." "I can't stand . . ."
2. *I cut the story off.* I like to imagine using a pair of golden scissors to snip it off close to my head.
3. *I find the feeling.* Immediately I turn my attention to

the feeling in the body that triggered the story in the first place. I notice where it is concentrated in the body, if it feels tight, loose, sinking, rising, hot, cold, etc. I focus on that sensation.

4. *I name the feeling.* "This is sadness/fear/shame/rage/hatred/frustration."

5. *I picture the feeling rising up like a wave.* I let the feeling get bigger, perhaps much bigger. I have learned I can let my whole body clench in rage, shake in fear, let my gut contract fully, let the pain in my heart be fully felt.

6. *I picture myself diving into the wave,* burrowing into it, swimming right down into the core of it. I keep allowing the feeling to deepen and intensify . . .

7. *I feel the wave peak and begin to die down.* I stay in the core, just paying attention.

8. *I feel myself open into what is here now.* As the feeling disappears, I notice what is here after the wave has come and gone. I open and expand into this calm, smooth ocean of peace, well-being and joyful tranquility.

The fourth is a decision-making tool, a way to let the deeper wisdom, not just this thin skin of surface consciousness, guide my actions. Here's what I do:

1. *I get still*, let my mind come to neutral and turn my attention to the body, especially the gut. I let it settle.

2. *I say,"I intend to _____ (Possible action A)."* I notice if the gut feels relaxed (a yes) or tenses up (a no).

3. *I let the gut settle again*, coming back to neutral.

4. *I say, "I intend to* _____ *(Possible action B)," * or perhaps just *"I do NOT intend to do A."* Again, I notice if the gut feels relaxed or clenches.

5. Then, *I have to believe my gut!* And I have found that invariably I can trust this internal yes/no: the body does not lie. When I have gone ahead despite an inner clenching, I have regretted it. When I have waited, something better, deeper, more profoundly miraculous has always shown up. And when I have taken action following a "yes" signal, the end result has always caused rejoicing.

Robyn Johnston:

I don't look back with any regrets. There is nothing that I want to do over. I look only to what is here right now. *The question I ask myself every day upon awakening is, "What's here? What is true for me this day?"* (That may change tomorrow, so I always take time to tune in!)

I also ask, *"If I were to go against the grain today, and do something totally unexpected, what would that be?"*

Susan D'Agostino:

To stay on my path, I *meditate and spend time alone.*

I continue to *allow the emotions to flow through* as they do and to *stay focused on what I DO want in my life.* Once a *week I trade Journey sessions with another practitioner.* I want to keep myself as clear as possible so I can keep living in each moment just as I AM.

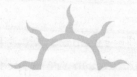

Authors and Contact Details

Here, collected for your convenience, are the brief synopses of each author's qualifications, specialties and contact information. All these practitioners and coaches would be delighted to connect with you and carry this conversation further. Feel free to contact any one of us; we welcome your questions.

Arsene and Kimberly Tootoosis are both founders of Red Echo Associates and work together as therapists and trainers. They provide workshops and trainings to First Nation/Indigenous communities and have worked in the field of healing and wellness since 1983. They can be reached at 306-398-4746 or 306-441-0725.

Bet Diening-Weatherston, her husband, Cam, and two sons, Jorin and Connor, live in a self-built timber-frame home in the rain forests of British Columbia's Sunshine Coast. Bet is a presenter for both The Journey and Visionary Leadership. She is also the Journey Workshop Coordina-

tor for North America. Visit her website at www.wouldyou
bewilling.com.

Cynde Sawyer and her husband, Mike, live as empty-nesters in the Chicagoland area in a rural, peaceful setting; their
children are now thriving as successful adults. Her hobby is
ceramics, which gives her a creative outlet that she did not
know she had earlier in life. Cynde has a passion to see people get beyond the beliefs that are holding them back from
a life of freedom, happiness and love. She is an internationally Accredited Journey Practitioner personally trained by
Brandon Bays, has been trained as an NLP Practitioner and
is a Licensed Spiritual Health Coach. She integrates all the
different processes to help clients gain freedom. Cynde can
be reached via email at cynde@thevisionaryway.com or at
www.thevisionaryway.com.

Debbie Clarke lives in Toronto and is an Accredited Journey Practitioner and Visionary Leadership Coach. She has
spent the past few years focusing on her own healing. An
important aspect of this healing has been to support Journey and Visionary Leadership work across Canada. Debbie
can be contacted at debbieclarke5075@sympatico.ca.

Jared and Ilene Beal are happily married (fourteen
years) and reside in Salem, Utah, with their five children,
five cats, twenty-one chickens, and one dog. Jared is running a bulldozer and loader at the local landfill, where he is
creating a recycling program. Ilene is a full-time mom. She

manages to squeeze in Journey processes and hosts two to three teleconference calls a month. Family comes first these days. Jared and Ilene enjoy planning family activities so they can spend more time together as a family. Their family motto is "The Family That Works Together, Plays Together, Stays Together Forever."

Jasmine Iwaszkiewicz is a practicing Accredited Journey Practitioner, Intuitive Energy Medicine Practitioner, Life Guide, Facilitator, Teacher and Healer who offers one-on-one sessions in person and via telephone. Jasmine facilitates workshops on Relationships and LIFE: Love, Integrity, Freedom & Empowerment. Contact her at Jasmine@TheAcademyofLife.com.

Joe Doyle and his wife, Nancy, also a Journey Practitioner, live in southern Virginia. Joe is a former business executive who served as an infantryman in the United States Marine Corps and is a veteran of the Vietnam War. He was eyewitness to the events of 9/11 in New York City. This tragedy brought the realization that trauma and conflict are not limited to just military veterans; we all suffer from post-traumatic stress. PTS is a wounding of the soul, not a disorder, and we store each wounding in our repressed cell memories. Joe can be reached by email at marinegrunt2@hotmail.com.

Lesley Strutt's work with The Journey and Visionary Leadership grew out of her own experience of unhealthy stress and disempowerment at work. Her near nervous breakdown led her to realize that feeling powerless can lead to ill health and deep unhappiness, and her journey to wellness and confidence created a desire to share with others the tools she uses. As a Journey Practitioner and a Conscious Coach, her passion is to help people become conscious of the choices they make in life and access their true potential no matter what challenges they face. Contact Lesley at lesley@lesleystrutt.ca.

Lori Beaty is an artist, entrepreneur, visionary, Conscious Coach and writer. She is passionate about cultivating creativity in herself and others using a wide array of integrated tools including Journey and Visionary Leadership processes, Non Personal Awareness (NPA), artistic awareness and development and shamanic healing practices. Lori is a regular presenter on Nightly Healing teleconference calls and is currently the president of Journey Outreach in North America. She offers both creativity and mandala workshops. Her coaching practice welcomes all who desire to flourish their creativity, heal creative blocks and raise their vibration through creative practices. You can follow her creativity coaching blog at www.clearlycreativecoaching.com or email her at lori@clearlycreativecoaching.com. You can also view her mandala art at www.collectivesource mandalas.com.

Lumananda and Bodhi Brouillette are internationally Accredited Journey Practitioners. Bodhi is also a certified Visionary Leadership Coach. They are owners of Live-n-Truth out of Boulder, Colorado, specializing in the process of helping others find and release limiting beliefs that have caused physical, emotional and mental suffering. For more information please go to www.liventruth.com.

Patricia Kendall is an Accredited Journey Practitioner, Certified Conscious Coach, and Licensed Spiritual Health Coach. Canadian by birth, American by residence, she takes great joy in supporting Journey Practitioners throughout this continent as co-founder and current president of the North American Journey Practitioners' Association. Pat's Journey practice welcomes all who seek healing, with a focus on survivors of childhood abuse; she also loves to assist healers of all kinds. You can visit her websites at www .lifepathconsulting.com and www.journeyforhealers.com or email her at patkendall@lifepathconsulting.com. Pat shares the beauty of northern Colorado with her partner, Beth, their four cats and her delightful Colorado Journey family.

Robyn Rae Johnston is a Nebraska cowgirl who enjoys wearing a variety of "hats" such as Accredited Journey Practitioner, Licensed Spiritual Health Coach, Professional Feng Shui Consultant and librarian. Robyn's joy in life and her ability to help others see new perspectives are shared through her writing, teaching, speaking and personal sessions. When not riding her horse, tending a garden or gathering eggs, Robyn loves spending time with her family hiking, biking, camping or golfing (basically anything to be outside!). She can be reached via email at cre8tivecowgirl@ gmail.com. Her website is www.open2awareness.com.

Susan D'Agostino resides in British Columbia, Canada. She is an Accredited Journey Practitioner, Certified Conscious Coach, Health Coach and Emotional Freedom Technique (EFT) Practitioner. Susan specializes in working with cancer patients and those suffering from depression and anger issues. She teaches EFT at the integrated cancer clinic in Vancouver, BC. Her book *Hello Susan, It's Me, Cancer!* was written after healing from breast cancer using alternative and natural therapies and is available from her website at www.healingeverybody.com.

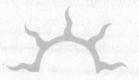

In Gratitude

With all my heart I would like to thank all the Journey Practitioners around the world who have offered their lives up to Truth, who've become a living transmission of grace, letting themselves be used by life in service to awakening and healing. I bow to the love that you are and to the extraordinary, life-changing work you do. Thank you, thank you, thank you.

I would also like to thank all the contributors to this book. I am blown away by your openness, your naked honesty and your willingness, for the sake of serving life, to expose your healing journeys in such a real, heart-opening way. I am awed and humbled by your stories, your love and the healing grace you are living in.

To Pat Kendall I offer a deep, deep Namaste of gratitude. Without you, Pat, this book would never have come together, and I stand in awe of the gargantuan labor of love it must have taken to birth such a beautiful, grace-filled book. And to Lesley Strutt, Pat's coeditor: you have such an exquisite way with words, such an elegant editing style. Thank you both. You are both editors in grace.

To my executive assistant Jo, I thank you for your dogged determination in hanging in there with me through the many hours spent in the creative fire and the long ten- to twelve-hour days of editing with me. It wouldn't have come together without you.

Kevin, I always feel I owe such a deep debt of gratitude to you for your thorough, carefully considered and thought-through copy edits in the days leading up to placing the manuscript in our publishers' hands.

And to our publishers everywhere, I thank you with all my heart for championing the work, and to Atria for getting the ball rolling on *Living The Journey*. To Michael Goerden, our German publisher, I always feel privileged and graced by your love of The Journey, your support of the work and by the depth of our friendship. Thank you!

To the Journey team in all the offices around the world, thank you, thank you, thank you! You are the heart, soul and embrace for this life-transforming work and a constant steady support for all those souls embarking on their journeys. I am so grateful to you all and would like to especially thank: Gaby, Cliff, Jo, Jane, Tricia, Debs, Claire and everyone else in the European office. Thanks to Katrina, Megan and all in the Australian office. Skip and Kris, you have been the mainstay for such a big continent in the North America office. People in Canada and America have been so very blessed to have you as the North American embrace. Also deep thanks to Lydia and John in the South Africa Journey office—your Journey Outreach work there is a wonder to me. Thank you all.

I would also like to thank our grace-filled presenters who have been offering Journeywork and advanced programs around the world: Debs, Bettina, Arianne, Anna Eva, Yvonne, Maarten, Skip, Bob, Marie-Sylvie, Annette, Ginny, Katrina, Laurie, Bill, Tamsyn, Sharon, Sayaka, Lydia and John. You are all a living expression of Truth. Life is blessed to have your service, and The Journey is graced to have you as both champions of the work and living expressions of it.

I would also like to thank Kevin again, this time in his role as CEO of The Journey and Visionary Leadership Program. I can't begin to tell you what it means to me to have my life partner standing alongside me offering this powerful healing work to the world. Thank you with all my heart for sharing this vision to bring awakening and healing to our planet. I pray it finds its way into every household so we can all find our way home to the beauty and grace within.

And a big debt of gratitude is owed to the teachers who not only inspired me but in whose presence freedom was realized. There are too many to list, but I would like to single out Gurumayi for that initial awakening. Also Gangaji and Ramana Maharishi for wordlessly guiding me to Papaji's feet, so he could smash the pot of the separate identity I had bought into. Every day with all my heart, Papaji, I thank you for the all-consuming grace that burns away the unessential, leaving me soaring in this love. My heart is forever bowed in gratitude to you.

And finally, deep gratitude to life itself for the extraordinary healing grace pervading life, embracing and supporting everything. May this life be lived in a never-ending prayer of gratitude to this infinite grace.

Namaste to you all.